RATIONAL

HOSPITAL PSYCHIATRY:

The Reactive Environment

RATIONAL HOSPITAL PSYCHIATRY:

The Reactive Environment

Jerrold S. Maxmen, M.D.
Gary J. Tucker, M.D.
Michael D. LeBow, Ph.D.

Dartmouth Medical School

Brunner/Mazel, Inc.
New York

published by
BRUNNER/MAZEL, INC.
64 University Place
New York, N. Y. 10003

Library of Congress Catalog Card No. 73-87723
SBN 87630-085-9

MANUFACTURED IN THE UNITED STATES OF AMERICA

FOREWORD

OUR IDYLLIC ROMANCE with hospital psychiatry came to an end in the sixties with the sad realization that institutional care, even the best kind, cannot eradicate mental illnesses. This disillusionment, along with the recognition that patients confined to institutions were—to an unparalleled extent—deprived of their rights and civil liberties, soon led to the conviction that hospitalization tends to be used by psychiatrists and society primarily for controlling undesirable behavior and is of dubious benefit to the mentally ill.

As might be expected, our inability to correct excesses in hospital practices by fine tuning soon produced other problems. In no time heroic efforts got underway to do all one could to avoid the evils of hospitalization—crisis intervention units sprang up; day and night and weekend hospitals became very popular; and even homes were converted into temporary asylums. As a result, even after severe illnesses psychiatric patients are today forced to re-enter an essentially non-supportive community, allegedly capable of resuming their lives as soon as their acute symptoms subside. Furthermore, a steadily increasing number of chronically ill patients are discharged after years of hospitalization, many of whom end up roaming our streets, sleeping on benches, and eating out of garbage cans, all in the name of freedom and right for self-determination.

Our new zeal also led to a blatant disregard of such conventional measures of treatment efficacy as low relapse rate and resumption of productivity. Institutions today are vigorously competing with each other by reporting shorter and shorter hospital stays.

Insurance commissioners and representatives of other third-party players have joined the choir with enthusiasm, insisting that hospitalization under all circumstances must be brief.

In this climate of appealing but oversimplified solutions, lack of data, and inadequate planning, it comes as a solace to read an objective presentation of the opportunities and limitations of hospital care.

Rational Hospital Psychiatry deserves the title chosen by its authors. Controversial issues are presented with enviable conceptual clarity, and though the authors clearly state their own views and preferences in the best academic tradition, the ultimate judgment is left to the reader. It is particularly refreshing to observe the sense of commitment with which the authors pursue the now unpopular notion that exemplary patient care cannot exist without deep commitment to continuous evaluation of our practices and devotion to continuous education of health professionals. Superbly organized and entertainingly written, this is the most comprehensive text that is available on this subject, and should be consulted by everyone who wants to learn about inpatient care from the perspective of a dispassionate and competent clinician. I put down this excellent book admitting that I wished I would have written it.

I only recently had the pleasure of meeting Dr. LeBow, but two of the authors, Dr. Maxmen and Dr. Tucker, worked with me for many years. I had the privilege of being their teacher when they began their careers in psychiatry and I could take a certain fatherly pride in seeing their accomplishments. Being somewhat of a cynic, however, I shall merely claim credit for having predicted that both of them would become outstanding members of the community of academic psychiatrists.

THOMAS P. DETRE, M.D.
*Chairman, Department of Psychiatry,
University of Pittsburgh
Director, Western Psychiatric
Institute and Clinic
Pittsburgh, Pennsylvania*

CONTENTS

Foreword by Thomas P. Detre, M.D. v

Preface xi

PART I: PSYCHIATRIC HOSPITALS: PAST, PRESENT,
AND FUTURE...1

1. Confidence Versus Despair: The Perennial Dilemma of
   Hospital Psychiatry 3
   A Brief History of the American Psychiatric Hospital 5
   The Era of Confinement 5
   Moral Treatment 7
   The State Hospital Era 10
   Biological Era 13
   Enter Psychoanalysis 15
   The Social Psychiatry Era 17

2. A Typology of Psychiatric Hospital Units 21
   Two Major Criteria 22
   Length of Stay 23
   Primary Treatment Modality 24
   A Typology of Psychiatric Hospital Units 26

3. The Reactive Environment 33
   Behavior as the Focus of Treatment 36
   Tailoring Treatment 40
   Sources of Change: Staff and Patients 43

vii

PART II: TYPES OF REACTIVE HOSPITAL ENVIRONMENTS...47

4. Crisis Intervention 49

5. The Therapeutic Community 57
   Treatment Program 60
   The Patient Sector 60
   The Patient-Staff Interface 62
   The Staff Sector 66
   Basic Principles of a Therapeutic Community.................... 69
   Bridging the Two Cultures.. 73
   Authority Relationships within a Therapeutic
   Community 74

6. The Token Economy 78
   Some Examples of Token Systems.................................... 81
   Terms and Meanings 85
   Observing and Recording Patients' Behaviors 91
   Tokens: What They Are and Why They Are Employed.... 96
   Techniques Used in the Token Economy.......................... 100
   Reinforcing Staff Performance 105
   Behavioristic Foundations of Token Economy Programs ... 108
   Is vs. Does Statements.. 108
   Measurable Products 109
   Deprivation 110
   Control 111

PART III: SPECIFIC PROCEDURES IN A REACTIVE ENVIRONMENT...115

7. The Admission Process 117
   Factors Affecting Psychiatric Hospital Admission.............. 118
   Admission Criteria 120
   Goals of Admission Procedures.. 123

8. The Hospital as a System.. 126
   Goals of a Hospital System.. 127
   The Use of Specific Treatment Modalities 129
   Disruptions of the System.. 131
   Acting-up 132
   The "Special Patient" Syndrome....................................... 135

9. Individual Procedures: Psychotherapy and Behavior
   Modification 139

Psychotherapy 140
Behavior Modification Programs 144

10. The Use of Medications in a Psychiatric Hospital.................. 151
    Guideline 1: All Hospital Staff Must Be Familiar with
      the Use of Medication... 152
    Guideline 2: Drugs Should Only Be Used When Properly
      Indicated; Conversely, They Should Not Be Withheld
      When Indicated ....:............ 153
    Guideline 3: Staff Attitudes Towards Medication Can
      Influence a Patient's Clinical Response..................... 155
    Guideline 4: The Use of Psychotropic Agents Should, as
      Much as Possible, Become a Collaborative Venture
      Between the Staff and the Patient................................ 156
    Guideline 5: During Hospitalization the Staff Must Try
      to Identify Those Patients Who Are Currently Not
      Taking Their Medication and Actively Find Ways to
      Prevent This from Continuing 159
    Guideline 6: During Hospitalization the Staff Must Try
      To Identify Those Patients Who Are Unlikely To
      Take Their Drugs Following Discharge and Actively
      Discover Methods to Prevent This from Occurring.... 164

11. Activities Therapy 167
    Functions of Activities Programs.............................. 168
    Diagnostic Functions 168
    Therapeutic Functions 170
    Abuses of Activities Therapy 173

12. Group Techniques 177
    Unique Qualities of Hospital Groups........................... 178
    Group Psychotherapy 179
    Staffless Groups 186
    Task Groups 187
    Role-Playing and Psychodrama 188

13. Family Involvement 191
    Information Gathering 193
    Family Therapy in a Psychiatric Hospital...................... 197
    Nuclear Family Therapy 198
    Multiple Family Group Therapy............................... 201
    Family Participation in Aftercare Planning................... 204

14. Planning for Aftercare 209
    Principles of Aftercare Planning 210
        Environmental Issues for the Discharged Patient............ 210
        Planning for Professional Outpatient Therapy................ 217
    Aftercare Programs 219

PART IV: ADDITIONAL PREREQUISITES OF A
REACTIVE ENVIRONMENT ... 223

15. Training, Research, Evaluation, and Record Keeping.......... 225
    Training Staff 226
        Staff Sensitivity Training 228
    Record Keeping 232
        Problem-Oriented Record 233
        Standardized Inter-Connected Data Collection Systems.. 236
    Research and Evaluation.. 237

Appendix A: Constitution of the Patient Advisory Board............. 245

Appendix B. Group Therapy Information....................................... 257

Bibliography 261

Index 275

TABLES

I.   Demographic and Diagnostic Characteristics of
        Tompkins-I 59

II.   "The Ladder System".. 61

III.   Sample Advisory Board Minutes 64

IV.   Typical Patient Schedule on Tompkins-I............................ 67

V.   Intervention Procedures for Producing and for
        Strengthening Behavior 103

VI.   Intervention Procedures for Weakening Behavior............ 105

VII.   Reasons for Hospitalization 121

VIII.   Sample Problem List.. 234

IX.   Sample Initial Plan 234

PREFACE

IN THE PAST fifteen years those who work in psychiatric hospitals have become inundated with a diversity of unintegrated theories and techniques. In fact we have reached a state where almost anything new is automatically embraced and implemented by hospital personnel without serious reflection or examination. This book has been written with the hope of providing the mental health professional with an integrated theoretical and practical approach to the hospitalized psychiatric patient. Instead of presenting a compendium of unrelated new techniques, we suggest a conceptual framework that synthesizes what we have found to be effective and rational treatment for psychiatric inpatients.

This conceptualization, which we have termed "the reactive environment," provides a framework that can be applied in many types of psychiatric hospitals, regardless of treatment orientation, patient population, or average length of stay. There has been no attempt to consider other types of therapeutic facilities, such as half-way houses, drug treatment centers, or day hospitals. Nevertheless, we believe the reader will find that the principles of a reactive environment are readily applicable to these other treatment settings.

This book is designed to be useful for everyone who works with psychiatric inpatients; for it is our contention that the notion of a reactive environment may offer new comprehensive guidelines for all those concerned with the care of hospitalized individuals.

This book is divided into four parts. The first part discusses the history of American psychiatric hospitals and offers a typology of contemporary inpatient facilities. It culminates with the most critical chapter in the book—a presentation of the principles of a reactive environment. Part II describes how these principles can be applied within the framework of three different types of unit-wide programs: namely, a crisis intervention unit, a therapeutic community, and a token economy. Part III elucidates how specific treatment techniques can be used most effectively in the rehabilitation of psychiatric inpatients. It discusses the admission process, the hospital as a system, individual psychotherapy, behavior modification, the use of medication, activities, group, and family therapy, as well as aftercare planning. In focusing upon these techniques we have deliberately avoided a "how to do it" approach, but rather have illustrated how the tenants of a reactive environment can maximize the effective use of these methods for hospitalized individuals. Finally, in keeping with the generic orientation of the book, part IV examines the role of teaching, research, evaluation, and record keeping within the psychiatric hospital.

The concepts presented in this book represent a distillation of many ideas derived from teachers, co-workers, and patients. To say thank you in print to each of these individuals would be a formidable task. But we especially would like to express our appreciation to Amy Aaron, Etsuko Inselburg, Kristi Kistler, Jenny Littlewood, and Nicky Nielsen for reviewing selected portions of this book. Furthermore, we would like to acknowledge Dr. Peter Whybrow who both encouraged us to write this book and facilitated our efforts in accomplishing this task. We would also like to thank Mimi Maxmen for her editorial assistance, as well as Joy DenHartog, Helen Harding, Jean Ollis, and Mary Smith for their secretarial contributions.

JERROLD S. MAXMEN
GARY J. TUCKER
MICHAEL D. LEBOW

Hanover, New Hampshire

Part I

PSYCHIATRIC HOSPITALS: PAST, PRESENT, AND FUTURE

IN 1970 ALONE 600,000 Americans were admitted to psychiatric hospitals (Hospitals 1971). The extensive range of experiences encountered by these patients is based upon theories and practices derived from the long history of hospital psychiatry. Nevertheless, as part I will document, contemporary hospitals are undergoing dramatic changes. Chapter 1 provides an overview of the history of American psychiatric inpatient treatment, demonstrating its alternating periods of idealistic progress and pessimistic stagnation. Chapter 2 presents a concise classification system of modern-day inpatient units that reflects the wide range of theoretical principles and treatment modalities currently being employed. Chapter 3 outlines what we believe should be the general theoretical framework for all forms of inpatient care—the "reactive environment." The principles embodied in this concept are central to this book, and represent a distillation of the most promising ideas of the future.

Chapter 1

CONFIDENCE VERSUS DESPAIR: THE PERENNIAL DILEMMA OF HOSPITAL PSYCHIATRY

AT A RECENT MEETING of the American Psychiatric Association several hundred psychiatrists were apparently listening to a series of erudite papers on the recent advances in hospital psychiatry. The "real" and unspoken agenda of the session, however, was the feelings aroused by about twenty protestors surrounding the meeting hall with signs that read, "hospitals are concentration camps" and "abolish psychiatric hospitals." While some of the assembled psychiatrists ignored those who were picketing, others seemed mildly unsettled by the content of the protest. For the experience only served to resurrect their own doubts regarding the efficacy and humanism of psychiatric hospitalization.

In no way could these doubts represent an isolated moment of reflection stimulated solely by a small band of malcontents. Those who work in psychiatric hospitals are continually having their fundamental assumptions and basic procedures attacked in the popular, academic, and even psychiatric literature. The popularity of *One Flew Over The Cuckoo's Nest, Titicut Follies,* and *Marat/Sade* suggests that these doubts strike a responsive chord in many. Goffman's analysis of total institutions in which he views the hospitalized patient as a helpless victim inextricably caught within an impersonal and dehumanized environment (Goffman 1961) has provided a scholarly impetus to this more generalized popular assault on the institution of the psychiatric hospital. Other writers have concentrated criticism toward the always vulnerable state hospitals (Deutsch 1948, Greenblatt 1955, Belknap 1956). Even among psychiatrists there have been those, like Szasz (1961) and Laing (1967), who by questioning the underlying assumptions of the notion of mental illness have condemned many of the common therapeutic regimens of contemporary psychiatric hospitals. Some have even suggested their abolition (Mendel 1968). Although the vast majority of American psychiatrists may readily dismiss the substance of these criticisms, they do seem to share with these critics an essentially similar attitude toward psychiatric hospitalization: namely, that hospitals are fundamentally miserable places to be in and that they should be utilized only under the most desperate of circumstances (F. A. Lewis 1962, Querido 1965). Given this perspective, it is of little wonder that those assembled at the American Psychiatric Association meeting were unsettled by the protestors' signs. To some degree these psychiatrists, although feeling a basic commitment to the idea of the psychiatric hospital, nevertheless had many of the same reservations.

In a sense, therefore, the meeting served as a microcosm of the paradoxical situation that these psychiatrists were experiencing. On the one hand, they, like the protestors, doubted the efficacy and humanism of hospital treatment; but on the other hand they were simultaneously excited to learn about the recent developments in hospital psychiatry. Indeed in the last fifteen years the field of mental health has witnessed the introduction of effective psychotropic drugs, the therapeutic community concept, group and family therapy, token economies, sophisticated aftercare facilities, and a whole mixture of differing forms of psychiatric hospitalization. All in all these recent innovations are giving rise to a new found optimism among those who work in psychiatric facilities. It seems therefore, paradoxical, but nevertheless all too apparent, that the contemporary psychiatrist experiences an upsurge of confidence as he learns about these new developments, while at the same time sensing a degree of despair as he listens to the afore-mentioned criticisms.

These coexisting, yet contradictory, feelings are not new to those concerned about psychiatric hospitalization. The entire history of American psychiatric hospitals reflects this ambivalence. In reviewing the past one cannot help but be struck by the alternating periods of confidence and despair that have hallmarked the historical evolution of the psychiatric hospital. In order to illustrate this it might be worthwhile to briefly recapitulate the history of the American psychiatric hospital. There are, of course, other reasons for doing so; for in large measure our current theories and techniques represent a distillation of this tradition. Furthermore, we can learn from such a concise history, since not all that is good in hospital psychiatry is new, nor all that is bad, old.

A BRIEF HISTORY OF THE AMERICAN PSYCHIATRIC HOSPITAL

The Era of Confinement

The precursor of the American mental hospital was the jail; it was here that the dangerous and not so dangerous deviant was confined. His incarceration, however, usually lasted for only a brief period of time. Since the prevailing Calvinist doctrine emphasized the immutable depravity of man, any attempt at rehabilitation was seen as an exercise in futility. Furthermore, there was rarely any problem finding a suitable "disposition," since exile from the community was a readily available solution (Rothman 1971). The proto-patient would then wander to another village until a similar series of events would be re-enacted. If perchance the deviant should commit the mistake of getting into the hair of the same community twice, alternate "solutions" could be implemented. For example, the "New England System" allowed hard pressed villagers to raise funds by auctioning their "lunatiks" to the highest bidder. As a result, the town accumulated wealth, the purchaser possessed a relatively inexpensive "slave," and the lunatic finally had a dwelling. In this way almost everybody was satisfied (Deutsch 1949).

With the passage of time work houses were established as repositories of the poor and feeble, demented and delusional. The work house was intended to "suppress and punish Rogues, Vagabonds, and common beggars" (Rothman 1971). Thus, in colonial America the mentally ill and the poor were incarcerated together. The only differential treatment was afforded those particularly troublesome lunatics who were sequestered in special cellar dungeons (Hamilton 1944). Such "treatment" received its justification from the prevailing "wild beast" theory of insanity. In short it was believed that lunacy resulted from the individual's submission to his lower animal instincts, and that only by inflicting pain could the individual be returned to his senses. The "wild beast" theory also provided the basis for the belief that the insane were insensitive to cold and thereby could readily tolerate the unheated dungeons in which they were incarcerated (Bockoven 1957).

Of even greater importance than the work house was the almshouse (or poor house), since for more than a century it sheltered the majority of the mentally ill. It was here that lunatics, impoverished beggars, wanderers, and other public nuisances were all crowded together in diseased infested rooms. In many ways the almshouse was similar to the work house, except that it would not admit those who had broken the law and, therefore, probably had a less objectionable clientele (Hamilton 1944). It was different, however, in a more significant respect. Whereas the *raison d'être* of the work house was punishment, the almshouse was intended to shelter, feed, and employ the poor. So convenient was this method of institutionalization that by 1840 there were 180 such facilities in Massachusetts alone (Rothman 1971).

As often seems to be the case, the poor received a different quality of care from that afforded the wealthy. Not unlike today, however, the treatment of the rich, although more genteel and costly, may not necessarily have been as effective. By the time of the American revolution the majority of well-to-do patients were treated according to Benjamin Rush's theories of mental illness. In essence he believed that insanity was largely due to congestion of the cerebral blood vessels and, as a result, prescribed liberal venesection, low salt diets, drastic purges, and all too effective emetics (Malamud 1944). Although the wealthy were "fortunate" enough to have these treatments administered to them at home, a few were hospitalized. In fact in 1752 the Pennsylvania Hospital became the first medical facility in America to have a separate unit for the emotionally disturbed. It was here that patients submitted to having their bodies chained, scalps shaved, and bowels purged in what nowadays may seem like bizarre methods by which to restore someone's emotional stability. With such indelicate forms of therapy it may be difficult to visualize this hospital as representing a progressive milestone in the history of American psychiatry. Yet, it was here that the practice of psychiatry was first introduced into a general medical hospital setting. Furthermore, at least in principle, it also was the first time in America that a public institution actively attempted to treat instead of merely to contain the mentally ill. Although by contemporary standards their methods appear sadistic, they still represented the best treatment that colonial medicine had to offer (Deutsch 1949).

Moral Treatment

Until the middle of the 19th Century the almshouse continued to be the main referral source for the mentally ill. Nevertheless, a few asylums were established that were devoted exclusively to the care of the emotionally disturbed. The first was founded in the 1770's in Williamsburg, Virginia, where the brutal treatment methods approximated those of the Pennsylvania Hospital (Deutsch 1949). Whereas initially these active "therapeutic" techniques were viewed as the potential remedy for mental illness, in time the enthusiasm of its practitioners diminished. In the process a fierce debate began to emerge over the value of physically restraining patients. Those who favored restraints felt they were necessary in order to prevent violent outbursts on the part of potentially disruptive patients. On the other hand the opponents argued that restraints demoralized the patient and encouraged regressive behavior.

In any event by the second decade of the 19th century there emerged a new idealism and humanism in American psychiatry. Borrowing from the reformative theories and practices of European's Pinel and Tuke, several corporate and state asylums established centers of moral treatment. At the outset it was the Hartford Retreat, the Worcester State Hospital, and the Bloomingdale Asylum that pioneered this trend. All of them combined a mixture of enlightened Calvinism and Quakerism sprinkled with some Yankee inventiveness and pragmatism to yield a cohesive, rational, and effective treatment system for the insane (Clark 1971).

Moral treatment did not represent any particular technique, such as non-restraint, but instead was a comprehensive approach to a patient and his aberrant behavior. By this approach the insane were admitted to an asylum where the alienist (i.e. superintendent) would provide parental concern over all aspects of the patient's life. Initially, the alienist would gather a history from the patient and his relatives, and then would proceed to diagnose his condition. After this was accomplished, the patient would be placed in a specific environment according to his particular emotional state. Thus, the "frantic, filthy, obscene, and profane" would be housed with those with a similar disposition, while the "melancholic and suicidal" would be situated "in view of cheerful scenery." As a result, the establishment of an individualized therapeutic program became one of the significant innovations of moral treatment. The alienist would relate to the patient as a responsible human being by encouraging him to suppress his abnormal behavior as well as to maintain self-control through the use of pledges and religious instructions. With kindness and firmness he would engage the patient in structured activities that simulated routine living situations. Another important characteristic of moral treatment was its disinclination toward utilizing restraints, whether they be physical or chemical (Clark 1971). Thus, in some way, the therapeutic program resembled what would now be considered to be milieu treatment, as well as incorporating, albeit in an unsystematized way, some contemporary principles of behavior therapy (Agras 1972a).

The advent of moral therapy had an immediate and profound impact on American psychiatry. Whereas previously, it generally had been felt that "once insane, always insane," enthusiastic claims of success suddenly emanated from the practitioners of moral treatment (Deutsch 1949). In 1832 Horace Mann reflected the spirit of unrestrained optimism by noting that, "Until the period comparatively recent insanity has been deemed as an incurable disease ... (However) it is now abundantly demonstrated that with appropriate medical and moral treatment insanity yields with more readiness than ordinary disease" (Report of the Commissioners Appointed to Superintend the Erection of a Lunatic Hospital in Worcester 1832). With complete solemnity wild claims of 75% to 100% cures were proclaimed, which were in fact gross distortions of the truth. Nevertheless, as a result of such extravagant pronouncements, a "cult of curability" reigned until the end of the 19th century (Deutsch 1949).

This unbridled optimism, however, led to the eventual demise of moral treatment. At best, these fabrications were intended to hasten the establishment of more enlightened psychiatric institutions, but at worst they were meant to enhance the reputation of the alienist. Regardless of the motivations behind these exaggerated claims, they tended to undermine the public's confidence in moral treatment so that whatever positive value it did possess was readily discounted by an understandably skeptical citizenry. There were other ways by which the alleged success of moral treatment led to its eventual downfall. As its popularity rose, the public finances necessary to support this rapidly growing venture became inadequate. As a result, overcrowded patients were tended to by overburdened staffs. With the quality of care degenerating, the insane were exposed once again to a custodial rather than curative experience. To make matters even worse the public reverted to the 18th century practice of institutionalizing the poor together with the insane. Alarmed by the massive immigration of Irishmen in the middle third of the last century, a frightened society used the asylum as a way of contending with "foreign, insane pauperism." In brief many Eastern states found it convenient to dispose of the Irish poor in particular by committing them to asylums, rather than to confront the underlying social and political problems raised by their presence (Commission on Lunacy 1855).

But even with all these problems it is possible that American psychiatry could, with strong leadership, have extricated itself from these numerous and complex dilemmas. Unfortunately, by 1850 most of the innovators of moral treatment had died without training individuals to carry on this tradition. Indeed this oversight may have been the greatest failure of the alienist (Bockoven 1963). Thus, once again, what had originated in a confident spirit of optimism and hope, eventually degenerated into failure and despair.

The State Hospital Era

Moral treatment was significant because at its finest it represented an idealistic and humanistic approach to the treatment of the mentally ill. Even at the zenith of its popularity, however, the vast majority of patients were still receiving custodial care in poor houses. Buoyed up by the "curability craze," Dorothea Dix, as well as other reformers, crusaded throughout the nation urging state governments to empty the almshouses and to assume full moral and financial responsibility for the treatment of the mentally ill. Eventually, with the support of the medical profession as well as the lay public, state governments established a series of large hospitals isolated from population centers whose task it was to treat those with emotional disorders. While there was general agreement on the need for such institutions, there was very little consensus as to whom they should treat and how they should operate. Some, led by a contingent from Wisconsin, urged that acute patients be treated actively in state hospitals, while chronic patients receive custodial care in county facilities. In the first place they argued that such a *county care plan* was more economical for the state. Secondly, by relieving the state hospital of the responsibility for custodial care they felt state institutions would then be able to concentrate their efforts on the active treatment of the acutely disturbed. And finally, it was pointed out that by occupying county facilities chronic patients would be closer to their families, have more employment opportunities, and be able to live in smaller institutions among a more homogeneous population of inmates. Opposed to this plan were professionals from New York who advocated a system of *state care,* whereby all patients, acute or chronic, would be treated in state hospitals. The major thrust of their argument was that the county care plan was based primarily on economic rather than therapeutic considerations. The generally inferior physician associated with county institutions, as well as the almshouse-like quality that prevailed within them, was contrasted to the superior medical services and the beautiful surroundings of the state hospital. Furthermore, those who advocated the state care plan felt that the gigantic size of the state hospital, rather than being a drawback, permitted better patient classification, provided more diversity in medical services, and facilitated a more efficient administrative organization (Deutsch 1949).

When considering the debate over county versus state care, one cannot help but feel that the origins of the aroused passions were more economic and political than philosophic and therapeutic. The whole controversy over administrative issues seemed to reflect a preoccupation with *where* rather than *how* patients should be treated. Occasionally, we get the unsettling feeling that our present day machinations over catchment areas resembles this 19th century debate over political and economic considerations.

Whereas in moral treatment the patient was perceived as an unique individual with specific needs, in the overcrowded state hospital he was viewed as an anonymous member of a throng. His only right was to be kept alive—not out of any sense of enlightened Christianity, but rather out of a legal necessity. Beyond his right to life all other rights were denied him. *En masse* patients were ordered to their beds, to their meals and to their day rooms where they were required to sit in stoney silence. Although misinterpreted, Darwin's *Origin of the Species* was used as an intellectual justification for this malignant regimentation of the insane. Since it was believed that mental illness was one of nature's methods for eliminating the unfit, effective and humane treatment was deemed unnecessary and undesirable. Accompanying this position was the prevailing medical view that mental illness was caused by an irreversible degeneration of the brain. Therefore, not only was successful treatment felt to be inadvisable, but impossible as well (Bockoven 1957).

In a sense the state hospital's allegiance to medical doctrine became even more peculiar, in that one of the unfortunate side-effects of the emerging state hospital system was its isolation of psychiatric care from the mainstream of the medical profession. As a result, whatever minimal spirit of scientific curiosity that did exist among physicians failed to stimulate the alienist's quest for a greater understanding of the etiology and treatment of mental disorders. At the end of the 19th century Dr. S. Weir Mitchell castigated hospital superintendents for isolating themselves from the medical profession, for failing to conduct research, and for misinforming the public as to the dangerousness of the mentally ill. He went on to accuse them of mismanaging their institutions, lacking interest in training psychiatric personnel, and possessing a generally complacent attitude toward their work (Mitchell 1894). Although his criticisms may have been somewhat overstated, there could be little doubt about the essential truth in his remarks.

Despite these deficiencies certain innovations were gradually being developed. In 1882 Dr. Edward Cowles established the first psychiatric nursing program at the MacLean Hospital (Malamud 1944). With the impetus of Dr. Adolph Myers' emphasis on the patient's total environment, social workers collaborated with psychiatrists to obtain a fuller portrait of a patient's family and community life. The necessity of such information became apparent, as discharged patients were increasingly unable to readjust to normal community life. Uncertain as to their own emotional stability and often having to confront a new living situation, the discharged patient was forced to contend with poverty, unemployment, and the "stigma of insanity." In order to alleviate some of these difficulties social workers, psychiatrists, and neurologists collaborated to establish aftercare facilities (Deutsch 1949), which eventually gave rise to ambulatory services. In spite of these developments it generally was felt that psychological intervention was of little utility, since insanity was believed to be the result of unknown biological forces; and it was these biological forces that increasingly gained the attention of the psychiatric profession.

Biological Era

Several factors coalesced at the beginning of this century to usher in the biological era of hospital psychiatry. The emergence of psychopathic hospitals facilitated a rapprochement between psychiatry and the mainstream of the medical profession. Affiliated with either university or general hospitals, institutions such as the Phipps Clinic (Imboden 1965) were usually situated in larger towns or cities. Modeling themselves after certain German institutions, they provided short term observation, examination, and treatment for acutely ill patients who were awaiting transfer to a state facility (Deutsch 1949).

Meanwhile, the organic etiology of some mental disorders was becoming increasingly apparent. The discovery of the spirochete responsible for syphilis, as well as the encephalitides which occurred during the 1917 influenza epidemic, demonstrated that microorganisms could be responsible for some cases of insanity. Similarly, advances in the understanding of vitamins, enzymes, and hormones led to the treatment of certain psychiatric disorders, such as pellagra, phenylketonuria, and cretinism. At the same time certain basic neuropsychiatric investigations, for example, those of Cushing and Penfield, illuminated the relationship between brain function and altered behavior.

Some physicians had anticipated that psychopharmacologic interventions would prove to be effective in alleviating, if not eventually curing, mental illness. In 1826 Balard's recognition that bromides frequently relieved excited patients ultimately led to its widespread and indiscriminate use among the general public. Thus, one hundred years after its discovery, one out of every five prescriptions was for some kind of bromide preparation (Alexander 1966). Hypnotics such as choral hydrate and barbiturates were also used, but had little effect on psychotic behavior, serving only to put the patient to sleep. In an attempt to relieve feelings of depression amphetamines were first introduced in the 1930's. Their transitory results and uncomfortable side-effects, however, rendered them of little practical use. Thus, pharmacologic intervention was, at least until 1954, of little value in the treatment of hospitalized patients.

In the meantime a number of discoveries were being made by European investigators. In 1933 insulin was given to schizophrenics, inducing a seizure, which was to be heralded as yet another cure for the dreaded disorder. Two years later the first frontal lobotomy was performed by Moniz and Lima which, although calming seriously agitated patients, frequently relegated them to the state of a minimally functioning robot. Cerletti and Bini in 1938 introduced the use of electroconvulsive therapy (ECT). Although initially employed in the treatment of schizophrenics, over the years it generally has been recognized as an effective treatment for "endogenous" depression, acute mania, and catatonic excitement. ECT grew in popularity to such an extent that by the 1950's it had become the most significant organic treatment in hospital psychiatry.

Despite these advances the care afforded patients in most hospitals remained primarily custodial. Although the stigma of emotional disturbances had been lessened and the importance of humane treatment generally had been recognized, it is, at least retrospectively, hard to get excited over labelling insanity "mental illness" and substituting straight jackets for padded cells. With inadequate staff and overcrowded conditions state hospitalization represented a frightening prospect for those in need of inpatient care. Even at the more expensive sanitoriums there was still little in the way of useful treatment. One only could hope that the natural course of the illness would eventually allow the patient to be discharged, and that the therapeutic machinations (or lack of them) of the staff would not impede this process. Even as late as 1952 a standard textbook of psychiatry recommends this treatment for the schizophrenic patient.

> "The patient, on admission, should be put to bed so that his behavior, his general bodily health and his sleep can be carefully supervised. The peace and quiet of a mental hospital, the orderliness and discipline, the tolerant and understanding attitude of those in charge, and the simplification of life, may at once produce a most gratifying change... The bodily health should be improved by good, nourishing food, and, when necessary, tube-feeding should be resorted to without undue delay. The bowels and bladder should be carefully regulated, and the skin made to act freely. Sleep must be promoted by open-air treatment, baths, warm drinks at night" (D. Henderson 1952, p. 337).

As can be seen, there was little in this therapeutic regimen that was not already utilized by the practitioners of moral treatment, despite the advances in biological psychiatry. Thus, at least until 1954, the early hopes that psychobiological research would yield major breakthroughs in the treatment of mental disorders had failed to come to fruition. Nevertheless, in comparison to the state hospital era the biological era of hospital psychiatry began to refocus attention on the actual treatment of patients rather than toward the quasi-political question of where they should be treated. And it is this development which remains the most important and enduring legacy of the biological era of hospital care.

Enter Psychoanalysis

As biologically oriented psychiatrists were slowly making

advances in the treatment of mental illness, psychoanalysis was rapidly capturing the imagination of American psychiatrists, intellectuals, and to some extent the public at large. So profound and pervasive was its influence that by the end of the Second World War it became (and may still be) the predominant force in American psychiatry. Its status was hardly undeserved, since it provided not only the first important comprehensive psychological theory of human personality and psychopathology, but also an innovative treatment technique and research instrument.

In the mid 1930's the Menninger brothers introduced psychoanalytic principles to the psychiatric hospital. Rather than merely viewing the sanitorium as an amiable place with ample amusements to pass the time of day, William Menninger suggested an individualized treatment approach in which the hospital would establish mechanisms for the expression of erotic and aggressive drives in a safe and socially acceptable manner (Menninger 1936).

Due to the reputation of the Menninger Clinic many of their prominent psychoanalysts were sought out in the postwar period by hospitals on the East coast. Establishing themselves at long-term facilities, such as the Yale Psychiatric Institute and the Austin Riggs Center, these analysts rapidly altered the nature of these institutions. Inspired by the work of Karl and William Menninger in Topeka and Harry Stack Sullivan and Frieda Fromm-Reichmann at Chestnut Lodge, psychoanalytic psychotherapy became the primary therapeutic modality (Kubie 1960, Rubenstein 1966).

Although these long-term psychoanalytic facilities could admit only a handful of patients and provide a therapy of debatable effectiveness at undebatably exorbitant costs, their impact should not be underestimated. For they generated a considerable amount of psychonalytic research and established the precedent of applying psychoanalytic psychotherapy to hospitalized patients; it is this latter effect that has largely contributed to the widespread application of insight-oriented psychotherapy in most of our contemporary psychiatric hospitals.

The Social Psychiatry Era

By the 1950's the proclivity towards any exclusive preoccupation with the patient's inner life was becoming increasingly suspect. Indeed, the importance of the patient's social environment was drawing greater attention from those in the field. To some extent this new direction was stimulated by certain psychoanalysts themselves, such as Harry Stack Sullivan (1931) with his emphasis on interpersonal relations and Theodore Lidz (1956) with his study of the schizophrenic family. Furthermore, psychoanalytic contributions to the rapidly developing field of group and family therapy increased the hospital psychiatrist's awareness of the patient's social environment. The most profound impact upon the psychiatric hospital, however, came not from the domain of the psychoanalyst, but rather from the efforts of British social psychiatrist Maxwell Jones. Working with patients who demonstrated severe social disorganization, Jones established in 1947 what was later to be called the "therapeutic community". Instead of the authoritarian, hierarchic structure traditionally associated with psychiatric hospitals, he promoted a system with egalitarian, permissive, democratic, and communal values. Everybody in the community, both staff and patients, was encouraged to maximize his therapeutic potential. Furthermore, all ward activities were deliberately integrated so as to be part of the total treatment program (Jones 1953).

In only a few years the therapeutic community notion found its way to this side of the Atlantic. Strengthened by the work of psychiatrists like Stanton and Schwartz (1954) and Wilmer (1958a) the therapeutic community concept spread so rapidly throughout the United States that no self-respecting hospital psychiatrist could publicly admit to *not* having a therapeutic community!

In an attempt to minimize the isolation of the psychiatric inpatient from his community there developed many other variations on the traditional hospital model. Sheltered workshops, halfway houses, three-quarter way houses, day and night hospitals all served to overcome the regressive tendencies of many hospitalized patients by keeping them within the community. At the same time a wide variety of inpatient settings, such as crisis intervention units, short-term hospitals, and long-term treatment facilities, was created in order to meet the specific needs of individual patients. Of equal importance was the application of behavior modification principles in the form of token economy systems for the treatment of chronically hospitalized individuals (Ayllon 1965). Thus, the social psychiatry era in hospital care introduced not only a multitude of differing treatment modalities, but also different hospital types.

Even though many advances were being made, most of them lay beyond the fiscal resources of the average American family. Besides documenting this fact, Hollingshead and Redlich (1958) also demonstrated that the economically disadvantaged were receiving inferior psychiatric treatment. These inequities led to the publication in 1961 of *Action for Mental Health,* which proposed the reorganization of psychiatric services in America. It pointed to the need for comprehensive community mental health centers and additional psychiatric units in general hospitals, which it was hoped would eventually render state hospital care obsolete. Two years later Congress implemented President Kennedy's National Mental Health Program, and, as a result, psychiatric inpatient units blossomed throughout the country.

As the number of psychiatric units in the general hospitals and community mental health centers increased, there developed a gradual reduction in the number of patients in the state hospital system. For example, in 1954 there were over 550,000 patients in state hospitals, while in 1970 the number was reduced by almost a third (New York Times 1972). Although in large measure this was due to the introduction of tranquilizers and anti-depressants in the 1950's, most psychiatrists would agree that the vigorous innovations in social psychiatry have contributed to this startling reduction in the state hospital population.

Underlying the community mental health movement has been

the fundamental assumption that hospitals should be resorted to only as a last ditch effort, and that every conceivable strategy should be used in order to maintain people within their community. Although laudable in spirit, this belief has possibly engendered a kind of phobic reaction to psychiatric hospitals. Flanked by certain literary and social critics, this quasi-ideological antipathy to the hospital among many contemporary psychiatrists has led to a devaluation of the potential benefits of inpatient care. Indeed it is ironic that in a period when the hospital is apparently more effective than ever before, it is possibly being viewed with more disfavor than at any other time in its history. In a sense it is this paradox that brings us back full circle to those ambivalent psychiatrists who observed the protest at their professional meeting. As they were encouraged by the new developments in hospital psychiatry, they were simultaneously doubting the hospital's effectiveness, humanism, or both. And it is living with this very paradox that has become one of the fundamental dilemmas for all reflective contemporary mental health workers.

In order to extricate ourselves from this dilemma we must avoid the pitfalls of those who have come before us. Unlike our forebears we should not confuse scientific innovation with scientific validation. At the same time we should not become sidetracked by a popular bandwagon of appealing slogans, such as "egalitarianism" and "humanism," *if* these slogans are devoid of meaning and substance, and only serve to justify a kind of therapeutic nihilism. If striving for "egalitarianism" really implies that we should minimize our clinical competencies, and if applying "humanistic" principles necessitates that we abandon the use of effective treatment modalities, such as behavior modification, medication, and psychotherapy, then we shall have abdicated our ethical responsibilities for patient care. Thus, if "abolishing psychiatric hospitals" would aid those suffering from emotional disorders, this book would represent nothing more than another anachronistic text contributing little to the already enormous body of psychiatric literature. We believe, however, that the psychiatric hospital still has an important place in the care of many emotionally disturbed individuals. Therefore, for us the question is not whether hospitals should exist, but *how* they should exist; that is, how they can best maximize their therapeutic potential. We feel that it is possible within a psychiatric hospital to begin restoring the patient to a productive life in the community by the application of critical scientific thought in concert with a fundamental respect for human dignity. It is to affirm this statement that this book has been written.

Chapter 2

A TYPOLOGY OF PSYCHIATRIC HOSPITAL UNITS

IN THE PRECEDING CHAPTER it was briefly mentioned that one of the recent significant innovations on the American hospital scene has been the emergence of a plethora of different types of inpatient units. Whereas only a generation ago there were basically two types of psychiatric hospitals, active treatment facilities and custodial care institutions, today there is a wide range of facilities offering radically different therapeutic programs. The developments that have contributed to this exponential rise in differing units have already been documented in the previous chapter. Further it is these same developments, especially the introduction of effective psychotropic agents, a greater awareness of the patient's environment, and the increasing costs of hospitalization, that have given rise to a second characteristic of contemporary psychiatric hospitals, namely, the trend toward shorter inpatient stays. Thus, whereas a generation ago a 90-day hospitalization was viewed as reasonably brief, today it would be seen as rather long.

As a result of these two developments, we feel that it would be valuable to arrive at a functionally useful classification of contemporary psychiatric hospital units. First, it would help to under-score that mental health workers can no longer view all psychiatric hospitals as having identical treatment goals, lengths of stay, and therapeutic programs. Second, it is necessary to distinguish among differing types of hospitals in order to arrive at the most appro-priate admission criteria. Since varying forms of inpatient care will provide different types of services, this distinction has prac-tical utility when it comes to matching particular patients with particular hospitals (Maxmen 1973b). Third, such a classification of psychiatric hospitals would assist in carefully defining some of the terms that will be used throughout this book.

We are basing our classification system of contemporary psy-chiatric inpatient facilities on our observations of and associations with many such units throughout the country. Because there is often a wide discrepancy between what therapists say they do and what they actually do, we have chosen to advance a typological system derived from what phenomenologically transpires on these units rather than from the particular slogans that are often used to describe them. It should be pointed out that this classification system establishes *general guidelines* rather than rigid criteria for differentiating psychiatric hospital units. Undoubtedly there are inpatient services that do not readily conform to any of these spe-cific categories and there are still others that would seem to con-tain elements of several hospital types. Nevertheless, from our experience we feel that this typology of psychiatric hospital units provides a functionally useful classification system that would apply to the majority of contemporary American psychiatric hos-pitals. Despite their importance, however, this typology of psy-chiatric inpatient facilities does not include alternatives to hospi-talization, such as drug treatment centers, half-way houses, etc. And finally, it should be clear that this typology reflects what we feel *does* exist, rather than what we feel *should* exist.

TWO MAJOR CRITERIA

Regardless of what a hospital staff espouses, the essential nature of their program is usually determined by the actual length of hospitalization and the unit's predominant treatment modality. We believe that these two parameters tell an observer more about how a psychiatric facility actually functions, than whether or not its ownership is public or private, its doors open or closed, its patients younger or older, its location urban or rural. Instead, by using the two criteria of *average length of patient stay* and *primary treatment modality* we feel we can advance a classification system of maximum utility and clarity. Although temporarily we shall discuss these two criteria separately, it should be recognized that to some degree these parameters affect one another. For example, a unit whose primary treatment modality is classical Freudian psychoanalysis, cannot effectively use this form of therapy with patients who are hospitalized for only a couple of days. Conversely, a crisis intervention model is, almost by definition, inappropriate for a long-term unit. Nevertheless, it is important to examine these two criteria separately in order to clarify terminology.

Length of Stay

We shall define the length of stay as the *mean* period of time a patient is hospitalized in a full day psychiatric service. A *short-term hospital* is one in which the mean patient stay is less than three weeks. An *intermediate-term hospital* is one in which the mean patient stay is between three weeks and six months. This type of facility is often called a "short-term hospital", because historically patients discharged in this period of time were considered to have had a relatively brief hospitalization. We would suggest, however, that in view of the recent emergence of many hospitals in which the mean patient stay is less than three weeks, it would seem anachronistic to speak of hospitalization greater than three weeks as being short-term. Therefore, throughout this book we shall refer to a hospital with the mean patient stay of three weeks to six months as an intermediate-term facility. And finally a *long-term hospital* is one in which the mean patient stay is greater than six months.

Primary Treatment Modality

By the primary treatment modality we mean that single technique which in reality is afforded the status of being the prime method for helping patients. In other words it is the form of treatment in which the staff *actually* invests its predominant therapeutic energies. Although most hospitals utilize a mixture of techniques, such as psychotherapy, medication, and recreation, generally speaking one treatment approach stands out; and it is this modality that will be considered of primary import. Finally, we do not wish to suggest that the primacy of a single treatment technique means that it is indeed the most effective, but only that either by choice or necessity it is the one in which the staff has the greatest investment.

Having said this, we feel that contemporary psychiatric hospitals emphasize one of the following seven treatment modalities:

1. *Crisis Intervention.* Derived from the conceptualizations of Lindemann (1944), Caplan (1964), and others, crisis intervention has become a general treatment approach directed toward alleviating the patient's acute stress resulting from a sudden alteration in one's social or biological systems. Broadly speaking, crisis intervention involves identifying this sudden change and rapidly intervening with a variety of techniques in order to quickly restore the patient to the mental state he possessed just prior to the acute change.

2. *Supportive Psychotherapy.* (see below)

3. *Psychoanalytic Psychotherapy.* In defining these two therapeutic treatment modalities it is easier to discuss them together, since in many respects the differences between them are more quantitative than qualitative. Regardless of its forms, psychotherapy can be defined as a psychological process between two people in

which the therapist by virtue of his position, training, and knowledge systematically attempts to apply mainly through verbal interchange certain psychological principles and techniques in order to modify the inner experiences, mental functioning, and overt behavior of the patient (Dewald 1964). In contrast to supportive psychotherapy psychoanalysis places a greater stress on transference, resistance, dream interpretation, and early childhood experiences. Psychoanalytic psychotherapy requires a longer duration of treatment and a greater frequency of interviews. The patient is more inclined to free associate and the therapist is usually less verbal. Its goal generally is a fundamental reorganization and reintegration of the individual's personality structure, given his innate talents and abilities. On the other hand supportive psychotherapy tends to rely on empathy, guidance, support, and reasoning in order to equip the patient for dealing more effectively with real life situations.

4. *Therapeutic Community.* This treatment approach was originally conceived by T. F. Main and became popularized by Maxwell Jones (1953) and others. Since then, the term "therapeutic community" has been used synonymously with other phrases, such as milieu treatment, administrative therapy, social psychiatry, sociotherapy, psychotherapeutic community, etc. As a result, programs that are called "therapeutic communities" oftentimes vary substantially from one another. Henceforth, a therapeutic community will be defined as a treatment modality which attempts not only to utilize maximally the therapeutic potential of the entire staff, but also to place a major responsibility upon patients to serve as change agents. In other words the unit's structure facilitates patients having a significant therapeutic role in the rehabilitation of other patients. Thus, all staff and patients meaningfully participate in the unit's decision-making processes about patient care as well as in the implementation of these plans.

5. *Token Economy.* A token economy is a treatment modality

that systematically applies the principles derived from general-experimental psychology, in particular, operant learning. It seeks to strengthen the patient's desirable behaviors and weaken his socially maladaptive ones by utilizing tokens as tangible and serviceable intermediaries between the patient's desirable activities and the positive reinforcers that are available to him. For example, a withdrawn patient may receive tokens for socializing with other patients, which he can then exchange for privileges or commodities he desires, such as watching television.

6. *Organic Therapies.* Essentially these refer to the use either of electro-convulsive therapy or of psychotropic medications which for the most part consist of phenothiazines, anti-depressants and lithium.

7. *Custodial Care.* Unlike the above, which are treatment approaches, custodial care will be defined as a method for keeping a patient alive and safe from physical or medical harm within the confines of a psychiatric hospital.

A TYPOLOGY OF PSYCHIATRIC HOSPITAL UNITS

By combining the two criteria of length of stay and primary treatment modality we can arrive at a classification of twelve types of psychiatric hospital units. In speaking about hospital *units,* rather than of hospitals *per se,* we are intentionally focusing on the functional components of these facilities that administer the treatment program, because some hospitals possess many different types of units. Once again, in presenting this typology we are attempting to classify hospital units according to what they actually do, rather than by what we feel they ought to do or by the official labels that staff may use to describe them. Thus, a hospital which primarily stresses psychoanalysis, but claims to be a therapeutic community because it has an occasional patient-staff meeting, would in this classification system be considered a type of psychoanalytic psychotherapy facility.

In describing these units we will speak of staff patient ratios, i.e. the total number of full-time professional staff, including nurses, social workers, psychiatrists, aides, etc., that generally work on these units in a 24-hour period. Arbitrarily, a staff-patient ratio of greater than 1:1 will be considered very high, 1:1-1½ high, 1:1½-3 medium, 1:3-10 low-medium, and less than 1:10 as low.

Furthermore, while there may indeed be other types of inpatient facilities, we feel these constitute the vast majority of those currently in operation. A brief description of the twelve types of psychiatric hospital units follows:

1. *Short-Term/Crisis Intervention.* In these units patients are hospitalized for less than three weeks in order to resolve some acute crisis or decompensation (Polak 1971, Lieb 1973). At some of these facilities the patient stay is set for a maximum of only three days (Weisman 1969). The task of treatment is usually to identify the precipitating stress that led to the acute decompensation and to intervene in such a way that the patient will be able to leave the unit as soon as possible. While in the hospital, no attempt is made to alter longstanding psychological difficulties. Medication and intensive individual and family therapy are usually the major treatment interventions. In order to accomplish this a high staff-patient ratio is generally required.

2. *Short-Term/Supportive Psychotherapy.* These facilities primarily offer supportive psychotherapy within a three week period. Unlike the short-term/crisis intervention unit there tends to be less organized activity so that at times it may give the outward appearance of being a "rest home" where patients can recuperate from the stresses of life. Although recreational, family, group, and chemotherapies may be available, they are of secondary importance to the psychotherapy between doctor and patient (Rosenzweig 1967). Generally speaking, the staff-patient ratio is in the medium range.

3. *Intermediate-Term/Supportive Psychotherapy.* In many re-

spects these hospital facilities resemble short-term/supportive psychotherapy units, except that patients stay between three weeks and six months (Linn 1955). Generally, the patients spend their day relaxing or participating in various low-keyed activities. The supportive psychotherapy is usually provided by the patient's outside therapist who visits on a more or less daily basis. In addition to this, group and organic therapies may be employed. Like other short-term hospitals, the goal is usually to have the patient function, albeit minimally, outside of the hospital. Usually the staff-patient ratio is in the medium range.

4. *Intermediate-Term/Psychoanalytic Psychotherapy.* These units provide intensive psychoanalytic psychotherapy to most of their patients in a period between three weeks and six months (Garber 1972). The goal of hospitalization is to resolve certain intrapsychic conflicts. It is assumed this will allow the patient to function outside the hospital. While some rudimentary attempts at a milieu program may be made, it is clearly of secondary importance to the dyadic relationship between the doctor and the patient. Outside of the formal psychotherapeutic hour the patient is usually relaxing or participating in some activity. Generally, little attention is paid to the patient's in-hospital behavior. Although medication may be used it is often done with great reluctance. So as not to interfere with the development of the transference, frequently the administrative details of a patient's program is under the auspices of a physician other than the one conducting the psychotherapy. The staff patient ratio generally lies in the high range.

6. *Long-Term/Psychoanalytic Psychotherapy.* Essentially, these facilities provide intensive psychoanalytic psychotherapy to generally quite disturbed patients in order to modify the individual's underlying personality structure (Menninger 1936, Caudill 1958, Rinsley 1968, and Gralnick 1969a). From six months to twenty or more years patients will be hospitalized, spending most of their day engaged in academic, occupational, or recreational activities. Although there may be some occasional patient-staff meetings, for

the most part the hospital structure is intentionally designed to facilitate the use of psychoanalytic psychotherapy (Edelson 1969). There is often a strong bias against the use of psychotropic medications, though on occasion they may be administered. In most instances the staff-patient ratio is in the high to very high range.

7. *Intermediate-Term/Therapeutic Community.* Unlike the aforementioned types of units the overall structure of the therapeutic community intentionally facilitates the patient's participation in and execution of the therapeutic program. It tends to place a primary emphasis on the total patient-staff community, rather than on the patient-doctor relationship (Kole 1966, Abroms 1969a, Almond 1971, L. H. Berman 1972b). The goal of such units frequently is to restore the patient to his optimal level of premorbid functioning, rather than to discharge him as rapidly as possible. In order to obtain these objectives the within-hospital behavior that occurs in a variety of large and small group settings is of paramount concern to staff and patients alike. Other treatment techniques, such as organic, family, and occupational therapies, may also be utilized. For the most part the staff-patient ratio is in the very high range.

8. *Long-Term/Therapeutic Community.* In many respects these facilities (M. Jones 1953, Whiteley 1970, Myers 1972) resemble those of their intermediate-term counterparts. The staff-patient ratio in a long-term therapeutic community is generally somewhat lower than in an intermediate-term facility, falling in the high-medium range. It should be pointed out that it is difficult to maintain a viable therapeutic community in a short-term facility (Raskin 1971). Although some practitioners feel otherwise (L. H. Berman 1972a, Greenley 1973), a short-term therapeutic community may not allow older patients to transmit to newer ones the norms, skills, and values that are essential for meaningful participation in such a program. In some respects many non-hospital treatment centers, such as half-way houses and drug treatment facilities, have a program that resembles a long-term/therapeutic community.

9. *Long-Term/Token Economy.* Unlike the facilities previ-

ously described, a token economy system systematically applies principles derived from general-experimental psychology, especially operant learning. In these units tokens serve as intermediaries between the patient's adaptive behaviors and rewards that are made available. Essentially, the patient receives a greater number of tokens for exhibiting increasingly useful activities, such as bedmaking, washing, etc. He can then exchange these tokens for desired privileges or activities, such as free time. Like the therapeutic community the patient's in-hospital behavior becomes the center of therapeutic attention (Ayllon 1968, Lloyd 1970). Medication, occupational, and recreational therapy may supplement this treatment regimen that for the most part has been used with chronically ill patients. The staff patient ratio is usually in the low-medium range.

10. *Intermediate-Term/Token Economy.* In many respects these programs (Hersen 1972) resemble those found in their long-term counterparts, except that the patients tend to be less regressed.

11. *Intermediate-Term/Organic Therapy.* In these facilities electro-convulsive therapy and medication constitute the major treatment techniques. Adjunctive group and supportive psychotherapy may also be used to a limited extent. For the most part the patient's day could be described as boring, consisting mainly of relaxation and recreation. The goal of treatment is to restore the patient so that he can function, albeit minimally, outside the hospital. The staff patient ratio is usually in the low range.

12. *Long-Term/Custodial Care.* Most frequently found in the state hospital system, these units provide custodial care for "hopeless" cases. The goal of hospitalization is merely to keep the patient alive by meeting his biological and medical requirements. No effort at rehabilitation is attempted with these patients who are disproportionately from the lower social and economic classes (Hollingshead 1958). For the most part these chronically ill patients demonstrate severe disorganization and regression, which

to a large degree is a concomitant of being institutionalized (Gruenberg 1967, Rosenberg 1970). The ward routines are incredibly dull and the milieu may at times resemble the proverbial "snake pit". Although occasional exceptions exist, patients usually become so dependent on these units that they are emotionally incapable of ever leaving them. The ratio of staff to patients is almost negligible.

That custodial units exist at all is a serious condemnation of American society, reflecting the persistence of the "wild beast" theory of insanity (Bockoven 1957), public apathy, and professional neglect. One cannot help but wonder how many human beings who could have otherwise been helped by alternative modes of treatment will be admitted *today* to such institutions. Hopefully, if the other eleven types of hospital units were sufficiently improved, we as a society would never have to resort to utilizing the twelfth.

By presenting this typology of psychiatric hospital units, we hope to illustrate that all hospitals cannot do everything equally well, and conversely, that certain units are better suited to achieve certain objectives. Since every geographical area has patients with varying demands, it is necessary, if these needs are to be met, that mental health workers have at their disposal a variety of different types of hospitals. All too often psychiatric inpatient facilities in the same locale establish programs that are nearly identical to one another. Instead, we believe it would be advisable that regional planning ensure that each geographical area possess a broad spectrum of psychiatric hospital units (Maxmen 1973b).

Even if such a network of inpatient facilities existed, we would not derive the full therapeutic potential that such hospitals would have to offer. Although a whole range of psychiatric units is necessary it is more important that the programs they offer meet the realistic needs of the individuals they serve. As suggested in chapter 1, it is not the existence of hospitals *per se*, but the quality of their programs that represents the difference between effective and humane treatment on the one hand and useless and degrading care on the other. Therefore, in chapter 3 we shall discuss those factors that can maximize the therapeutic potential of the psychiatric hospital, as well as present a theoretical framework for its operation.

Chapter 3

THE REACTIVE ENVIRONMENT

DESPITE THEIR DIVERSITY all contemporary psychiatric hospitals can be guided by the fundamental principles of what we shall call a "reactive environment."[1] These principles neither cast a psychiatric hospital into one specific mold nor delimit the range of effective treatment modalities that currently exist. Nevertheless, they constitute the essential elements of all forms of effective hospital care.

A reactive environment may be defined as one in which the unit's overall structure maximally utilizes and coordinates the entire staff's efforts towards the rehabilitation of the patient's particular behavior problems so that ultimately he becomes a longstanding and productive member of society. In such an environment the entire staff is primarily concerned with the patient's specific activities and responds to them in an integrated and consistent manner. In doing so it capitalizes upon the most unique aspect of the hospital setting which allows for interaction,

---

[1] The term "reactive environment" is drawn from Ferster's 1971 use of this concept in reference to psychotic children.

observation, and treatment of the patient on a twenty-four hour a day basis.

A reactive environment is in contrast to a psychiatric hospital in which the entire staff does not uniformly relate to a patient's specific behavior. Frequently, this is most apparent when the primary focus of treatment rests almost exclusively within the traditional doctor-patient relationship. Oftentimes this results in viewing the rest of the patient's activities in the hospital as being either of ancillary significance or of no importance at all. Therefore, this conceptualization fails to utilize the unique potential of the hospital's full day living situation and does not provide adequate treatment guidelines for those hospital personnel who are not privy to these doctor-patient contacts. Another factor that may render the hospital environment non-reactive is when its staff automatically relates to all patients with a set of previously established routines irrespective of an individual patient's special and current needs. In other words the hospital deals with all patients in the same manner and does not differentiate between the diverse treatment requirements of an individual patient. Furthermore, such a program does not vary its treatment regimen as the patient's therapeutic needs change during the course of hospitalization. Thus, a unit may be considered non-reactive if its staff fails to create conditions by which a flexible and consistent therapeutic focus on the patient's current behavior is maintained throughout his entire stay.

It is preferable to view the concept of a reactive environment as being on a continuum rather than being an all or nothing phenomenon. One could speak theoretically of 75% reactivity, 25% reactivity, etc. Ideally, an environment that is 100% reactive to a patient's needs is one in which *every moment* of the patient's hospital life is maximally utilized in order to bring him closer to regaining his status as a functioning member of society. An environment that is 0% reactive to a patient's requirements is one in which his adaptive strivings are underdeveloped or even prevented.[1]

Many factors can minimize the reactivity of the psychiatric hospital. Perhaps the most subtle one is when there is an unspoken or unrecognized diversity among hospital staff as to the goals of hospitalization. While some staff members may see the objectives of hospitalization as being achieved only when the patient has resolved specific psychodynamic conflicts, others may believe it is attained when he can "express his feelings"; still others may think it is accomplished when the patient no longer argues with the staff. At other times the hospital personnel may be striving toward incompatible objectives. For example, the social worker may encourage the parents to set firmer limits, while the psychiatrist may encourage the adolescent patient to liberate himself from parental domination. Some psychiatric hospitals maintain relatively nonreactive environments because the staff primarily attempts to serve its own needs, such as running the ward smoothly or being excessively preoccupied with their own sensitivity groups. And finally, a psychiatric hospital cannot become a truly reactive environment if its clinical care is determined more by the patient's economic status than by his treatment needs. Society as a whole must ensure that all its citizens can avail themselves of effective hospital treatment.

All psychiatric hospitals operate as temporary total environments for patients. As a result, the staff is aided in their treatment efforts by virtue of their complete or nearly complete control over both the critical antecedents and consequences of every one of the patient's behaviors. Herein lies the important and unique potential of psychiatric units for either their therapeutic or regressive effect. Hospitals can provide the patient with the encouragement and opportunity to behave adaptively or they can fail to develop or even inhibit this potential. Thus, to a large degree the hospitalized patient is a captive of an environment—beneficial, benign, or harmful—wherein his adaptive and, paradoxically, his unadaptive activity can be nurtured. Even his contacts with the outside

---

[1] Except where indicated, we will use the term reactive environment in the positive sense; that is, approximating 100%.

community can be regulated and titrated. Inherent in a hospital's overall structure must be mechanisms that will react to the patient's specific behaviors and encourage his adaptive strivings. This is not to say that a unit-wide program *per se* is antithetical to the patient's successful treatment or to the individualization of his care.

The principles governing the occurrence of adaptive and maladaptive activities are the same. Thus, one set of methods can strengthen both classes of behavior, while another set of techniques can be used to weaken them. Because the hospital personnel has control over most of the conditions affecting the patient's activity, the staff can use these principles to his benefit or to his detriment.

BEHAVIOR AS THE FOCUS OF TREATMENT

The practice of hospital psychiatry should, above all else, focus on the patient's *behavior*. This view does not imply behavior therapy in the colloquial sense, but does mean that therapy sets as its goal the diminution of the patient's specific maladaptive activities and the augmentation of his adaptive behaviors. We say this because it is a patient's behaviors that get him into the hospital (N. Jones 1965, J. J. Muller 1967), and it is a modification of these activities, as well as the acquisition of new competencies, that will allow him to successfully and permanently leave it (Tucker 1973).

By the term "behavior" we mean a patient's publicly observable verbal and non-verbal activity. Mental illness is a psycho-social-biological process which can give rise to some, although not all, forms of maladaptive behavior. Diagnostic categories of mental illness are useful to the extent that they provide an indication for possible pharmacological interventions and a clue to the patient's overall prognosis. Beyond that, however, we choose not to talk of mental illness or diagnostic syndromes, as they often conjure up other specific treatment techniques and may obscure that aspect of the patient's behavior that is causing him the most difficulty. We find it more useful to look for and focus upon the prominent symptoms or activities that seem to interfere with the patient's functioning, especially those bringing him into conflict with other people in his environment. By concentrating on behavior one can more readily delineate specific treatment plans and more accurately measure the extent of therapeutic progress.

We have found that most behavior problems can be divided into five broad categories (LeBow 1973).

1. Behaviors generally considered intolerable by society, regardless of their frequency, e.g. fire setting, incest, self-mutilation, etc.

2. Behaviors which become intolerable only if they occur too frequently, e.g. *always* complaining of aches and pains.

3. Normally acceptable behaviors which occur in inappropriate settings, e.g. laughing at a funeral.

4. Deficiencies in behaviors generally expected in a particular setting, e.g. mutism, failing to eat, etc.

5. Behavioral sequellae of unusual inner experiences that adversely affect the patient or those in his environment, e.g. hallucinatory behavior, delusional speech, etc.

As this classification system illustrates, deciding if a particular activity is maladaptive requires a consideration of not only the behavior *per se*, but also the *setting* in which it occurs and the *frequency* of its expression.

Although a behavioral focus does not necessarily negate the supposition that disordered activity reflects disturbances of psychic structures, it does not assume that in order to treat the behavior one has to change underlying psychological mechanisms. This view sharply contrasts to those held by many individuals who feel that permanent behavior change can only occur if there exists between the therapist and the patient a mutual psychodynamic understanding of the supposed "roots" of behavior. Even if one acknowledges the significance of unconscious motivation, it is not the unconscious, but rather the activity stemming from the unconscious that gets the patient into difficulties.

If treatment is to be based on the patient's behavior, then the model of hospital care that is most effective is one that orients its primary concerns around *pragmatic* questions of *rehabilitation*[1] rather than theoretical assumptions about how to "cure" mental illness or acquire "self-understanding." This is not meant to imply that a staff must divest itself of any theoretical position, but only that it should not let its preferred orientation prevent it from doing what may be helpful to the patient. Thus, if a therapist should find that phenothiazines lead to adaptive activities in a particular patient, then such treatment should be continued even though it may violate the therapist's theoretical preferences. By doing so it is hoped that the patient will survive whatever theoretical axe we have to grind.

Unfortunately, the treatment of hospitalized patients is all too often based upon etiologic theories of mental illness (e.g. Rubenstein 1966, Gralnick 1969b, Abroms 1971b). We do not eschew or negate the importance of etiologic searches for the origins of mental illness, but we do reject making etiologic formulations and speculations *the* necessary and sufficient data from which treatment decisions are made. For example, on the assumption that pathological family interactions give rise to schizophrenia, we do not believe, as some have (e.g. Abroms 1971b), that family therapy is necessarily indicated for the treatment of that disorder. In our view family therapy should be *used* only if there is a reasonable likelihood that it will be pragmatically effective in the patient's rehabilitation. Again, if we use the rehabilitation analogy, no one claims that the techniques of speech or physiotherapy are suitable for removing the vascular occlusion responsible for a stroke, or

---

[1] In a sense the term "rehabilitation" is more precise than "treatment" in that we propose a model of hospital practice that strives to return the patient to a higher level of functioning rather than to "cure him of his illness". For the sake of literary convenience in this book we will use the terms treatment and rehabilitation interchangeably. The term "cure" will only be used to connote the successful outcome of the entire treatment process. Because for the vast majority of inpatients hospitalization is but one phase in their overall rehabilitation, one cannot expect hospitalization to cure the patient; a cure can only result during the aftercare stage of treatment when the patient has successfully completed his rehabilitation.

that they would be effective in preventing future cerebral vascular accidents. Nevertheless, they are the major techniques for the rehabilitation of patients with these conditions. We are suggesting a *"non-etiological position"* only in the sense that to be useful a treatment does not have to be based on etiological theories, but only be effective in rehabilitating the patient's behavior problems (Tucker 1973).

We believe that some of the major difficulties in linking treatment with an etiological theory are as follows: (a) The treatment must then be consistent with the theory which may determine what can and cannot be treated. For example, Freud's early feelings about schizophrenia excluded this illness from the scope of psychoanalytic therapy. (b) A total commitment to any single etiological theory and its accompanying treatments limits the therapist's range of interventions. (c) The goals of therapy often become the fulfillment of a theory rather than what the patient actually needs or desires (Tucker 1973). Many therapists may object to this disassociation of etiology from treatment because it does not get down to the "cause" of the problem. The facts are, however, that we do not know the etiology of many psychiatric problems and even if we did, we may not have the appropriate techniques consistent with the etiology that would effectively alleviate the condition. Until both of these developments occur we have found it most helpful to base treatment decisions on what is pragmatically useful rather than theoretically speculated.

Utilizing treatment methods derived from pragmatic considerations requires a great deal of flexibility on the part of those who conduct therapy. Because staff all too often possess a limited repertoire of therapeutic skills, patients frequently continue to receive a particular treatment long after its ineffectiveness has become apparent. For example, if a patient has failed to improve on adequate doses of anti-depressants, it is ill-advised to maintain him on that drug merely because he continues to be depressed. In other words if a treatment does not work, change it. Because the hospital staff can provide careful observation throughout a twenty-four hour period, they have the opportunity to safely treat patients empirically, flexibly, and pragmatically.

TAILORING TREATMENT

In order to implement treatments based on pragmatic considerations it is necessary for the hospital to have available *many potentially therapeutic techniques* (Abroms 1969a, Tucker 1973). Whether these techniques include group therapy, behavior modification, psychodrama, chemotherapy, or whatever, it is important that they can be applied by a staff who is knowledgeable in their use. Furthermore, their employment should be *selective*, based upon the current and specific needs of individual patients. The indiscriminate use of *all* therapies for *all* patients is not tailoring treatment.

The concept of tailoring treatment implies more than simply establishing an individualized treatment plan. It also implies that staff constantly up-date, and, therefore, adjust their therapeutic efforts according to the patient's current behavior. Furthermore, tailoring treatment suggests that the techniques of specific therapeutic modalities may need modification, if they are to be utilized optimally in a psychiatric hospital. Oftentimes these changes are necessary because both the hospital setting and the characteristics of the patients admitted to it frequently contrast with those found in an outpatient facility. Unlike ambulatory patients hospitalized individuals are living together for twenty-four hours a day, and usually demonstrating a greater degree of behavioral impairment. Furthermore, the actions of one inpatient oftentimes affect the behavior of other ones. Because of these and other differences, certain treatment modalities require modification when applied to hospitalized individuals. For instance, whereas extra-group socialization oftentimes is discouraged in outpatient group psychotherapy, we believe that with hospitalized individuals it should be fostered. Further examples of such treatment modifications will be presented in part III.

In order to tailor treatment it is useful to have a multiplicity of therapeutic settings in order to evaluate how specific patients will behave in a variety of situations (Moos 1967, 1968). For example, patients may react one way during individual contacts and another way in a large group. Thus, to only observe a patient in a single treatment setting may deny the staff information that would become available only if the patient participated in a variety of situations. In fact one of the advantages of psychiatric hospitalization over outpatient care is that the patient can be exposed to a number of treatment settings and can be observed in a multiplicity of interpersonal situations.

Another requirement of a reactive environment in tailoring treatment is to consider whether the patient's within hospital activities will be useful to his post-hospital life. That is, the staff needs to ascertain if the behavior generated in the hospital will be adaptive in the many settings of the patient's future life. For example, although an inpatient may become better able to express his anger, if he does so at work he may endanger his job, since his boss in all likelihood will be less tolerant of this emotion than is the hospital staff. Indeed, to the extent that the patient is given the opportunity to acquire behavior that society judges to be important and to divest himself of activities that his particular culture judges to be offensive, psychiatric hospitalization becomes an effective and useful experience.

Furthermore, the patient's long-term adjustment in the community will be highly related not only to the activities he engages in or fails to engage in, but also to his becoming responsive to the consequences society typically administers for those behaviors. Thus, although the offering of praise for accomplishing essentially elementary tasks within the hospital may temporarily help to strengthen positive behavior, it is unlikely that the patient will receive the same rewards as often for similar tasks outside the hospital. In short the patient must learn to exhibit useful activities and to become responsive to the rewarding practices of his particular sub-culture. We are not proposing subjugation to the "system," but merely that the patient become aware of how his behavior interacts with the "system," either to his benefit or detriment. How the patient uses this information depends upon his goals and interests.

In a reactive environment effective treatment also requires that the patient's activities be made known to the entire treatment staff. Knowledge of what the patient has or has not been doing before he entered the hospital is essential for the designing and implementation of a treatment plan. More specifically, adequate assessment data detailing the patient's behaviors in regard to his peer, work, and family environments help to reveal his assets and deficiencies with respect to these surroundings and, thereby, help to set the occasion for implementing tailored treatments by the entire staff. Significant individuals in the patient's social matrix may be interviewed in order to provide a useful picture of the patient's morbid and pre-morbid functioning. Furthermore, these interviews may indicate the way they will respond to the patient's behaviors after leaving the hospital. Comprehensive evaluation of behavioral functioning, therefore, is a critical precursor of effective treatment.

Of course, the patient's own activities on the unit, especially his interactions with other patients and staff, continually provide extremely valuable assessment data. During the course of hospitalization this information can be utilized in order to modify and to up-date treatment plans. Thus, hospital programs need constant reevaluation so that they maintain their effectiveness in dealing with the patient's current behavioral repertoire. When a great disparity exists between the on-going hospital activities and the patient's present behavior, it is unlikely that much therapeutic progress will be achieved. To remedy this schism intermediate programs need to be instituted, whereby the patient can acquire the skills that will enable him to derive the full therapeutic benefits of the various hospital activities. For example, a functionally mute patient may need to be helped to speak at some minimal level before he can profit from group therapy. On a more general level it is essential in tailoring treatment that a patient possess a certain number of skills before he can acquire new behaviors in a particular hospital activity.

The concept of tailoring treatment should also be applied when preparing the patient for one of the most important tasks of a reactive environment, namely, aftercare preparations. Briefly, this task involves incorporating into the overall structure of the treatment program techniques that will increase the likelihood that the benefits derived from hospitalization will be sustained after discharge. The failure to do this may indeed be the greatest deficiency of contemporary psychiatric hospitals. Because many staffs generally have little to do with the post-hospital care of the patient, it would seem as if "out of sight, out of mind" is a prevailing theme in many facilities. A reactive hospital environment develops techniques that maximize efforts in helping patients successfully adjust and sustain themselves in the community.

SOURCES OF CHANGE: STAFF AND PATIENTS

Traditionally, patient care in a psychiatric hospital was determined exclusively by the psychiatrist, while other staff members merely functioned to execute his specific directives. Because of the influence of Maxwell Jones (1953), Stanton and Schwartz (1954), and others, the role of *all* staff increasingly became recognized as necessary in the effective functioning of the psychiatric hospital. Nevertheless, the traditional and autocratic medical dominance still persists, albeit in a somewhat more subtle form. Statements like "the patient always perceives the doctor as being the only vital figure in his treatment," or "ultimately, the physician has legal responsibility" have justified minimizing other staff's therapeutic involvement. A medical autocracy is ill-suited for a reactive hospital environment. In a relatively non-reactive hospital the sixty minutes between the patient and his psychiatrist is usually the center of therapy, resulting in a tendency to relegate the other twenty-three hours of the day to a lower level of importance. This contrasts with a reactive environment where the hour between the doctor and the patient should be considered no more crucial than any other hour.

As a result, all staff who interact with the patient during the day must play an equally important role in the planning and implementation of the overall treatment program. This total involvement is necessary so that the hospital personnel can share information, arrive at and execute a unified treatment plan, and assure that maladaptive behaviors are not being encouraged. Accomplishing these objectives may be inhibited unless the unit possesses a *full-time staff*. All too often outside psychiatrists who make brief daily visits to the hospital attempt to direct the patient's therapeutic program by "remote control." Similarly, other staff will have difficulty becoming fully acquainted with the patients and optimally equipped to respond to their everchanging needs unless they are full-time members of the treatment team. A system with part-time social workers, or nurses who rotate between medical and surgical services will provide less than ideal patient care.

In and of itself a full-time staff will be inadequate unless it is fully trained to carry out its assigned responsibilities. On-going teaching programs for all staff, not only psychiatrists, are valuable for enhancing their level of competency and for facilitating greater involvement with patients. Part of this educational process may also include an attempt on the part of hospital personnel to constantly evaluate its own therapeutic effectiveness by means of follow-up studies and staff discussions.

Staff will be unable to work consistently with one another unless the hospital's program provides for readily accessible avenues of communication. The major mechanisms by which this relevant information can be exchanged consist of frequent staff meetings and a concise and informative record keeping system. If unresolved intra-staff conflicts exist, others have suggested that these communication vehicles will be rendered inadequate and patient care will be compromised (Stanton 1954, Main 1957). In order to remedy this situation some have advocated the use of "staff sensitivity" sessions with the intent of alleviating intra-staff tension (Abroms 1969a, Sager 1972a). Although these meetings may have some occasional utility, they can become so absorbing for the participants that staff become preoccupied with their own behaviors rather than those of the patients.

Having stressed the importance of harnessing and utilizing the therapeutic expertise of all staff, we do not wish to imply that every staff member can or should do everything equally well. Varying staff have differing kinds of skills, knowledge, and experience. To ignore this reality by establishing a kind of "pseudo-egalitarianism" by which everybody does everything is to waste the potential resources of individual staff (Tucker 1973). A social worker who is particularly skilled in family therapy should concentrate on that area, rather than be encouraged to learn about and to administer, for example, psychological tests. Thus, individual staff members should concentrate on utilizing and extending the competencies they possess. Also, we should mention the importance of having a staff that is rewarded for their efforts. Too often it is merely taken for granted that staff are willing to extend themselves in order for the patients to get better. Patient improvement is not always a sufficient incentive for a staff's optimal efforts and, therefore, alternative methods for rewarding staff must be utilized.

Depending upon the type of psychiatric hospital unit the patients may, to a greater or lesser degree, also serve as valuable sources of information and assist in the rehabilitation process. The optimal use of patients as an integral part of the treatment program generally has been associated with intermediate and long-term therapeutic communities. Nevertheless, it has been demonstrated that patients may also play a useful, albeit less pervasive role in the rehabilitation of other patients in short-term units (Greenley 1973, Maxmen 1973a) as well as in token economies (Ludwig 1971). The degree that patients are incorporated as rehabilitative agents should be a reflection of the behaviors they possess that are relevant to the task at hand. At the same time, patient involvement should be directed toward the meaningful and constructive objectives of the hospital program. For example, to have patients spend excessive amounts of time deliberating over the decor of a hallway is of considerably less value than discussing and trying to modify another patient's maladaptive behaviors. Thus, patients in a reactive environment can be continually involved in a program that allows them to gradually increase their responsibility for one another (e.g. Fairweather 1964).

In summary we have suggested that because of its total or near total control over what patients do, the psychiatric hospital can create an overall structure that maximally utilizes and coordinates the entire staff's efforts towards the rehabilitation of patients' specific behavior. In this manner the staff should establish the conditions by which the patient ultimately may become a long-standing and productive member of society. Inherent in this proposal is that the practice of hospital psychiatry must capitalize on the important relationships existing between the patient's behavior and his environment. Among the specific recommendations set forth were that the psychiatric hospital staff adopt primarily a behavioral focus, pragmatically select treatments that fit the patient's individual needs, emphasize rehabilitative goals, and initiate meaningful aftercare arrangements early in the patient's treatment. We have also indicated the importance of involving family members, of having an educated staff which is rewarded for its efforts, and of utilizing varied therapeutic techniques. We wish to stress that the concept of a reactive environment may fit, to a varying degree, the operations of seemingly dissimilar psychiatric hospitals. Part II describes these possible applications.

Part II

TYPES OF REACTIVE
HOSPITAL ENVIRONMENTS

THE PRINCIPLES of a reactive environment may be applied to all forms of psychiatric hospitals, and may be integrated with other theoretical concepts of inpatient care. Part II illustrates these assertions. The next three chapters will outline, respectively, the general principles of hospital-based crisis intervention, therapeutic communities, and token economies. Specific examples are described, demonstrating how each unit incorporates the principles of a reactive environment. Certainly, many of the theories that will be enumerated may be incorporated into many types of psychiatric hospitals without adopting their more elaborate and complex structures. The particular units that are described represent approximate forms rather than ideal versions of reactive environments. Nevertheless, they provide us with some concrete examples of the direction we feel hospitals should take in order to optimally meet the needs of psychiatric inpatients.

Chapter 4

CRISIS INTERVENTION

FROM CONTEMPORARY USAGE it is not clear whether the term "crisis intervention" stands for a new treatment modality, a rationale for intervention in any life situation, or a legitimatization of any psychotherapeutic measure short of psychoanalysis (Schulberg 1968). But regardless of its definition the concept of crisis intervention has been utilized as a coherent framework for brief goal-oriented hospital treatment that emphasizes the promotion of adaptive behavior and follow up care. Crisis intervention implies a time-limited focus for both the conception of a problem and its treatment. This is in direct contrast to psychoanalytic practice in which the formulation and treatment of a problem requires an extended and ill-defined period of time. Unlike crisis theory, psychoanalysis views current emotional state as a summation of forces that have developed almost from the individual's intrauterine existence.

The clearest description of a crisis has been made by Caplan who defines it as when an "...individual is faced by stimuli which signal danger to a fundamental need satisfaction or awake major need appetite, and the circumstances are such that habitual problem-solving methods are unsuccessful within the time span of past expectations of success" (Caplan 1964, p. 39). Viewing an emotional crisis as an obstacle to important life goals places the crisis in a conceptual framework that allows the clinician to examine all aspects of the patient's life, in addition and often to the exclusion of intrapsychic dynamics. Through this theoretical framework the clinician can legitimately examine and modify the social matrix of the patient. No longer does the therapist need to feel that any intervention short of a complete restructuring of a person's total personality is invalid. Instead, psychiatric hospitalization can focus on resolving the patient's immediate crisis.

According to Caplan (1964) a crisis develops in four phases: (a) The individual experiences an initial elevation of tension or anxiety which summons customary or habitual homeostatic problem solving responses. (b) The tension continues to increase, the person becoming more upset and ineffectual due to continuation of the stimulus causing the situation plus a lack of success in resolving the problem. (c) The tension reaches a point where additional (internal and external) resources are mobilized to solve the difficulty, or the individual may turn away from the goal he was trying to attain. (d) If the problem cannot be satisfactorily resolved, the mounting tension may result in major disorganization and behavioral impairment. If the crisis is successfully resolved, however, this resolution can significantly enhance the individual's functioning so that he is often able to perform at a higher level than that prior to the crisis. Caplan also believes that with the proper type of psychiatric assistance an enduring positive change can often result from successful adaptive solutions to crisis situations.

With this theoretical background it is of interest to examine two hospital units that were designed to deal with crisis situations. One such facility was the Emergency Treatment Unit (ETU) of the Connecticut Mental Health Center that was started about 1968 in New Haven, Connecticut (Weisman 1969, Thomas 1970, Lieb 1973). The stated goal of the ETU was to "focus on current life struggles in order to facilitate the individual's return to the level of functioning preceding the disruption and crisis that led to hospitalization" (Weisman 1969). The setting of the open door unit was adjacent to the lobby of the mental health center. The patients used the lobby as a day room so that they would not have the feeling of being "put away." The unit had rooms for seven patients. Patient selection was limited to those who were acutely ill, had a history of functioning well immediately prior to their crisis, and whom the staff felt it could help. The staff used the following techniques in treatment:

1. *Time-limited contracts.* This consisted of an explicit statement to the patient before admission that he would only be hospitalized for a maximum of three days, followed by thirty days of outpatient treatment. This time-limited contract was believed to be important in promoting rapid identification of the problems by both the patient and the staff.

2. *Intensive intervention through multiple therapist teams.* There was a deliberate attempt to have the patient relate to the unit rather than to an individual therapist, thereby discouraging dependence on "the doctor". In order to achieve this objective the patient was seen daily by several staff members (mostly nurses and aides) who collectively shared the responsibility for his treatment. Furthermore the unit attempted to have a staff of mixed racial and ethnic backgrounds in order to hasten the development of a therapeutic rapport between minority group patients and members of the treatment team. The individual contacts of the staff were supplemented by several types of community meetings, group, and family therapy. In this manner the patient became familiar with many different therapists and treatment modalities. Although these multiple therapist contacts could continue during the outpatient phase of treatment, for the most part the patient was assigned to one member of the team.

The staff viewed the primary goals of treatment as maximizing the autonomy of the individual and focusing on the acquisition of adaptive behavior. The emphasis on autonomous functioning was particularly important; the staff felt that dependency was one of the cardinal symptoms of an unsatisfactorily resolved crisis. They attempted to deal with this by having the patient participate in most decisions about his care, as well as imposing few restrictions on his daily activities. The treatment dealt with some intrapsychic and interpersonal conflicts, but mainly concentrated on current life stresses, such as work, finances, family conflict, etc. The staff insisted that the patient focus on these stresses as directly as possible. The spirit of treatment could be summarized by the frequently asked question, "What are you going to do?"

Using these techniques of time-limited, goal-oriented therapy, the unit treated about 450 admissions yearly. Its patients did not differ from those admitted to other inpatient units, although they were predominately from lower social classes (Class 4 and 5, Hollingshead Scale). About 40% of the patients had previous hospitalizations and about half of these had an admission diagnosis of psychosis. Interestingly, the outcome statistics and readmission rates from this unit seemed no different from other longer term facilities (Weisman 1969).

Being situated in a large metropolitan area, the ETU was specifically designed to fulfill the emergency needs of an urban population. In establishing a "crisis unit" in a rural area, however, one must make certain modifications in the treatment program in order to meet the requirements of patients from small isolated communities. The conditions requiring these modifications are both numerous and complex, but two of them are of particular note. (a) Patients frequently come from long distances, usually without the aid of convenient transportation. (b) Generally, there is a relative paucity of psychiatric facilities either for inpatient or ambulatory care. Thus, because a rural psychiatric hospital may be the only one in a wide geographical area, it is especially important that its program maintain a high degree of flexibility in order to treat a great diversity of psychiatric patients. As a result of logistical difficulties, the telephone and two-way closed circuit television (Solow 1971) must occasionally replace face-to-face meetings between the hospital staff, the patient, and his relatives. Whereas in a metropolitan area patients can usually return for follow-up care to the institution in which the inpatient facility is located, in a rural setting this oftentimes becomes impossible. Instead, one frequently must use the ambulatory facilities within the patient's particular community. Although this usually has many advantages the available resources tend to be rather limited. As a result, follow-up is frequently conducted by local ministers, general practitioners, welfare case aides, etc.; and therefore, close liaison with them becomes an important task of the hospital staff. Thus, a rural psychiatric hospital must shape its program to meet the particular realities of non-urban life.

An example of such a facility is the Dartmouth-Hitchcock Mental Health Center (DHMHC) which is a 28 bed[1] adult short-term/crisis intervention unit affiliated with a general hospital and the Dartmouth Medical School. Located in rural New Hampshire, the unit frequently admits patients who must drive up to two or three hours in order to reach it. All patients are admitted on a voluntary basis and the unit maintains an open door policy. The patients themselves present with a wide variety of severe behavioral disturbances and stay on the average of 18 days (Maxmen 1973a). This latter figure can be somewhat misleading in that patients usually remain in the hospital anywhere from overnight to 30 days. Because of its training responsibilities, the unit possesses a high staff to patient ratio.

Prior to admission patients are screened by either psychiatrists in the community or by the walk-in service of the Dartmouth-Hitchcock Mental Health Center. On entering the unit all patients receive an intensive medical and psychological evaluation. This assessment procedure includes the administration by nurses of the Psychiatric Status Schedule (PSS) (Spitzer 1970) which measures specific behavioral indices (see chapter 15). The PSS

---

[1] In addition to the regular 28 beds, the unit also maintains two extra ones for patients who are admitted for a maximum of 48 hours. These two "emergency" beds are utilized as are those on the ETU in terms of time-limited contracts, specific admission criteria, etc.

helps the staff focus on specific areas of behavioral impairment and is used in follow-up investigations. To complete the initial assessment all family members are interviewed on the day the patient is admitted to the hospital.

In determining which of a multiplicity of treatment approaches are to be utilized with individual patients, the members of the staff convene bi-weekly in team meetings. It is here that assessment data is collected and treatment plans with specific time-limited goals are formulated. In order to enhance liaison activities the patient's outside therapists or social workers are frequently invited to these sessions.

Because of the unit's rapid patient turnover, it is vital that the entire staff keep abreast of current developments. For that reason a half hour staff meeting is held six mornings a week. These meetings are immediately followed by group therapy which allows therapists to see the majority of their patients almost at the outset of the day. Afterwards, depending upon the nature of the patient's behavioral disturbance, a wide variety of treatment modalities is available, including individual therapy, evening group therapy, psychodrama, family therapy, alcohol discussion groups, Alcoholics Anonymous, occupational counseling, recreational activities, E.C.T., pharmacotherapy, and individualized behavior modification programs. The availability of a wide diversity of treatment methods is important, especially in a rural area, because there are no other accessible inpatient facilities that can provide these therapeutic modalities.

The unit treats approximately 500 patients annually and demonstrates a recidivism rate lower than most longer term facilities. Although follow-up studies are conducted only a month after discharge, 85% of the patients show a marked degree of behavioral improvement.

Both of the above units operate on crisis intervention principles and, therefore, share many more similarities than differences. In addition both emphasize (a) time-limited contracts, (b) specific goals of treatment, (c) a rapid identification of the changes that led to the crisis, (d) a willingness to engage in various environmental manipulations, (e) a follow-up period of care, (f) an attempt to maximize the autonomy of the patient, and thereby minimize his dependency, and (g) an involvement of all people who are important in the patient's social matrix.

Many of these principles are those that we have enumerated as being the components of a reactive hospital environment. Furthermore, the results from these short-term settings are apparently similar to those found in longer term facilities (Caffey 1971). This latter finding may reflect that hospital treatment is seen as only one phase of the overall treatment program; the vast majority of rehabilitative efforts are carried out on an outpatient basis. In the ETU this is done by the unit's staff. In the DHMHC the staff continues with outpatient treatment whenever possible, but for the most part it arranges for and collaborates with other treatment agencies in the patient's local community.

Certainly, for most patients short-term/crisis intervention is able to restore the patient's functioning so that he can continue treatment on an ambulatory basis. Nevertheless, other patients may require continued hospitalization in longer term facilities. The next two chapters discuss the principles and techniques of two of these hospital types.

Chapter 5

THE THERAPEUTIC COMMUNITY

LIKE ANY SLOGAN, the "therapeutic community" can mean many things to many people. It would seem that for some psychiatrists it refers to a hospital setting in which an occasional group meeting is conducted in the presence of "home-like" furnishings. Yet for others (Sager 1972a) it implies a complete participatory democracy in which patients decide on all activities and treatment programs whether or not they possess the expertise to do so. From our own experience, most so-called "therapeutic communities" subject their patients to a random hodgepodge of activities ranging from intensive individual psychotherapy to basket weaving and basketball, the only overall guiding theoretical structure being provided by a schedule of these activities. These poorly reasoned almost non-programs have become all too common in American psychiatry. Part of the vagueness in the term "therapeutic community" lies in the phrase itself. Any collection of patients and staff can constitute a community, and nobody is going to say that their program is less than therapeutic (Pinsker 1966). Thus, as many authors have noted, the term therapeutic community is an ill-defined catchall phrase, greatly in need of both a theoretical framework and a meaningful definition (Wilmer 1958b, Pinsker 1966, Zeitlyn 1967, Abroms 1969a).

In chapter 2 we defined a therapeutic community as a type of psychiatric hospital unit which attempts not only to maximally utilize the therapeutic potential of the entire staff, but, more importantly, to place the major responsibility upon the patients themselves to serve as primary *change agents*. The therapeutic program is designed to facilitate patients having a significant role in the rehabilitation of themselves and other patients. A vehicle must be provided by which all staff and patients can participate in decision making processes about patient care and the implementation of these plans. Although historical data are utilized in arriving at a treatment plan, a necessary ingredient of a therapeutic community is that the in-hospital behavior of the patient is an important source of information for the treatment. For the sake of clarity let us reiterate that by our definition a therapeuic community is one form of a reactive environment, with most of its essential characteristics as outlined in chapter 3. What is specific to the therapeutic community, however, is that it emphasizes that the patients have a major role as change agents. In order to assure that this occurs, a therapeutic community needs a well-defined, coordinated, and structured program, so that almost any interpersonal situation in the hospital helps to transform the "patient" to "change agent".

What we are about to describe is one type of therapeutic community, namely, Tompkins-I (T-I). We have chosen it because two of us had a long-standing affiliation with the unit and one of us was its director for a number of years. The unit has received considerable attention and has been the subject of intensive research for more than a decade. Therefore, a discussion of its program can be bolstered with data. Finally, this unit has shown a considerable degree of effectiveness which gives credence to the potential benefits that can be derived from a therapeutic community.

Tompkins-I is a 28-bed acute psychiatric service in a general hospital (Yale-New Haven)[1], that was established by Dr. Thomas Detre in January of 1960 (Detre 1961a). Its patients have demographic and diagnostic characteristics as indicated on Table I (Harrow 1972). It should be noted that the unit accepts patients who for the most part demonstrate an inordinate amount of behav-

TABLE I

DEMOGRAPHIC AND DIAGNOSTIC CHARACTERISTICS OF TOMPKINS-I

AGE

12-19	29%
20-24	20%
25-34	20%
35-44	9%
45 and over	22%

SEX

Male	36%
Female	64%

EDUCATIONAL LEVEL

Did not graduate high school	27%
High school graduate	16%
Some education beyond high school	19%
College graduate	20%
Some education beyond college	18%

DIAGNOSIS

Schizophrenia	40%
Psychotic depression	12%
Neurotic depression	13%
Personality disorder	22%
Others	13%

NUMBER OF PREVIOUS HOSPITALIZATIONS

None	65%
One	20%
Two	8%
Three or more	7%

ioral impairment and cognitive disorganization. Because the average length of stay is approximately 62 days (Maxmen 1973c) economic realities favor the admission of middle and upper class

---

[1] Recently, the Tompkins-I program has been moved to a new facility called "10-East".

patients. Although most patients are admitted on a voluntary basis, a few are committed on an emergency certificate to the unit. For the most part it is open door facility, but it can be locked, if necessary. As a major unit of the Department of Psychiatry of the Yale Medical School, it has a very high staff patient ratio in order to carry out both its clinical program and training responsibilities. It should be noted that without its academic functions a lower staff patient ratio could adequately sustain the unit's clinical program.

TREATMENT PROGRAM

The actual structure of the unit can best be understood by describing three interrelated components of the program: (a) the patient sector, (b) the staff sector, and (c) the interface between the two.

The Patient Sector

The patient sector has several key aspects. The first of these is the "ladder system" which refers to a series of specific statuses assigned to each patient according to the level of "responsible" behavior he exhibits. The patient gradually moves up from the lowest "rung" of the ladder, where he has minimal responsibility and receives maximal surveillance, to the highest status, where he has relative autonomy and a great deal of responsibility. The ladder system is described in Table II. The particular status of each patient is determined by the second key component of the patient sector called the *advisory board*. As a kind of patient government, it deals with requests for status changes, home passes, and most other aspects of patient life in the hospital (see Appendix A). The advisory board meets at least three times a week with the entire patient community to consider, discuss, and vote upon written requests submitted by the patients. After thoroughly discussing the proposed patient status change, pass, or present unit problem

TABLE II

"THE LADDER SYSTEM"

Status (rung)	Description	Indications
Admission		
Staff-Special	Constant accompaniment by nurse.	High suicide or assaultive risk. Seriously confused. Can take minimal responsibility for self.
Patient-Special	Constant accompaniment by a member of the Monitor Pool (See below).	Less of a suicide or assaultive risk. Moderately confused. Can take some responsibility for self. Patients feel able to safely accompany him.
Ten-Minute Checks	Monitor Pool member contacts him every ten minutes.	No longer a suicide or assaultive risk. Minimal confusion. Some appropriate interpersonal involvement. More or less able to assume responsibility for his in-hospital behavior. Has begun to openly discuss problems.
Independent	Nobody accompanies the patient.	No confusion. Demonstrates a moderate level of appropriate interpersonal involvement. Able to assume full responsibility for his in-hospital behavior and can openly and spontaneously discuss problems.
Monitor Pool	The patient serves as a "specialer," "checker," and "monitor." As a specialer he accompanies other patients on patient-special and as a checker he contacts those on ten-minute checks. As a monitor he assists the staff in performing management and organizational functions on the unit.	Can initiate and maintain a high level of interpersonal involvement. Able to assume responsibility for others. Has memorized Monitor Pool rules. (see Appendix A).
Buddy System	Monitor Pool duties. May go outside of the hospital on walks and passes.	Has successfully functioned as a specialer, checker, and monitor at least once. Likely to take responsibility for self outside the hospital.
Discharge		

with the entire patient body, the advisory board votes on the particular issue. In reaching these determinations they can consult with members of the nursing and activities staff, but the final verdict is left to the patients. The board itself is led by officers selected by the patients.

Besides advisory board meetings, the patients have two other types of programs which are held without the presence of the staff: *big leaderless* and *little leaderless*. Both of these group sessions provide patients with an opportunity to share problems, exchange ideas, and provide feedback without the assistance of staff. Their major function is to tangibly convey the message that patients can serve as change agents without relying on professional assistance.

The Patient-Staff Interface

One way to view the organization of this unit is to see its structured activities and rules as serving regulatory functions. This regulation occurs at two levels. The first is the management of individual patient problems by staff and patients which attempt to promote adaptive behaviors and to minimize maladaptive ones. The second is the regulation of the overall patient community which seeks to maximize its effectiveness. These two forms of input are coordinated not only by the structured activities of the unit, but also by the staff clearly stating what it believes are adaptive and effective behavior. The regulatory activity of the staff is partially maintained through the exercise of clearly defined authority and through continued monitoring and feedback of patient behavior. Although the staff performs these functions throughout the day, they are implemented most explicitly during the formal patient-staff meetings. These sessions are extremely important for several reasons. They graphically convey to patients that their deliberations are taken seriously by the staff and that their decisions are usually competent and will be implemented. Furthermore, during these meetings the patients seem to use the staff's questions and statements as models for their own inquiries and therapeutic interventions. And finally, these sessions allow the staff to present clear guidelines as to what behaviors are deemed important for patient progress. These large community sessions are conducted by a staff member in a business-like manner with a specific agenda and time limitations. There are three such meetings during the week. The first is held Monday morning and consists of a weekend report presented by the patients. These reports systematically provide observations on all patients for the weekend with supplemental comments being offered, if necessary, by the staff. The other two weekly patient-staff meetings are structured around a mimeographed summary (prepared by the patients) of the previous advisory board meeting. These minutes list all requests for status changes and passes, specific patient problems and other general items for discussion (see Table III).

The staff leader opens the meeting by asking if anyone would like to bring up anything listed in the minutes. All status changes and pass requests not brought up are automatically implemented. Those that are raised for consideration are discussed and either approved or vetoed by the chairman. In reaching this decision the leader clearly states his reasons for so doing. Although a clear-cut consensus is desirable, at times this is not possible and the chairman has to arrive at an autocratic determination. Before doing so, he frequently asks for a sense of the meeting, but ultimately, the final judgment rests with him. On occasion, however, he postpones making a conclusion and refers it back to the advisory board, or to a future patient-staff meeting for further consideration. When disagreement persists between the staff and patient sectors, it is dealt with openly. Hopefully, divergent opinions can be reconciled, but if not, the presence of differing perspectives is acknowledged and freely commented upon. Acting-up behavior, however, is overtly discouraged by interrupting the present activity and immediately dealing with the disturbance. For example, a patient who did not like a decision made about his pass request

TABLE III

Patient-Staff Meeting—January 7, 1972

ADVISORY BOARD MEMBERS

Mrs. A. — Chairman	Mr. F.
Mr. B. — Vice Chairman	Mr. G.
Mr. C.	Mrs. H.
Miss D.	Mrs. I.
Mr. E.	Secretary: Mr. J.

STATUS REQUESTS

1. Mr. F. requests monitor pool.
   Vote: 5 yes, 4 no
2. Mr. K. requests patient-special.
   Vote: 9 yes, 0 no
3. Mr. L. requests independent status.
   Vote: 2 yes, 7 no
4. Mrs. A. requests a pleasure pass from Saturday, January 8th at 11:00 a.m. till Sunday, January 9th at 6:00 p.m.
   Vote: 6 yes, 3 no
5. Mr. M. requests buddy system.
   Vote: 6 yes, 3 no
6. Mr. E. requests a work pass on Saturday, January 8th from 11:00 a.m. to 4:00 p.m.
   Vote: 0 yes, 9 no
7. Mrs. N. requests ten-minute checks.
   Vote: 8 yes, 1 no

INFRACTIONS

1. Mr. G. failed to pick up his special.
   Decision: Verbal reprimand
2. Mrs. O. came in late twice from a buddy walk.
   Decision: Demote her to monitor pool

DISCUSSION ITEMS

1. The unit is a mess.
2. The patients feel uncomfortable around Mr. P. and are running out of patience.
3. The nurses are giving inaccurate reports.

got up and spat into a wastebasket. Various staff and patients asked him to take a seat and explain his behavior. Conversely, silent members of the group, particularly those who are able to participate, are commented upon and asked to join the discussion.

Our description of patient-staff meetings would not be complete without mentioning *emergency sessions*. These are convened in times of crisis by anyone, although usually by the staff, for such reasons as someone eloping from the unit, taking drugs, or fighting. In these situations the available staff responds immediately and decisively. Initially, a brief staff meeting is held as soon as possible after the event in order to inform the hospital personnel of what has transpired and to agree upon a tentative plan of action. This is immediately followed by an emergency patient-staff meeting attended by everyone, including the patient(s) most intimately involved in the crisis. The meeting serves several purposes: (a) It acknowledges that a most unusual event has occurred and that it is necessary to discuss it. (b) Further information is sought and shared with all those in attendance. In most crises it becomes apparent that more than one person is involved or has information in advance about the disturbance and fails to tell anyone. (c) A distinction between "squealing" and information-sharing which might prevent a crisis is discussed and emphasized. This is especially important for adolescents for whom drug use on or off the unit or impulsive running away are distinct possibilities. (d) By sharing information patients and staff can attenuate the escalation of potential rumors. (e) The values of the unit are reiterated with the strong message that Tompkins-I "is a hospital and not a jail," and that such behavior is totally "unacceptable." (f) The final purpose of the emergency patient-staff sessions is to reach a concrete resolution of the acute problem.

Whereas routine patient-staff and emergency meetings have a more or less "executive" format, the other kinds of sessions where staff and patients interact can be considered to have a more classical therapeutic function. These include individual, group, fam-

ily, and multiple family therapies as depicted in Table IV. In
these sessions as well as in the patient-staff meetings the bulk of
individualized treatment plans are implemented. For example,
although the vast majority of patients attend group therapy, the
leaders may choose to encourage assertive behavior in a withdrawn
patient, but discourage it in an overly aggressive one.

The Staff Sector

The staff meets by itself in essentially two types of sessions.
The first consists of small *team meetings* and the second of large
staff meetings. The staff is divided into four teams which meet on
a bi-weekly basis. Each team consists of a senior staff member, a
psychiatric resident, several nurses, a psychiatric social worker,
and an occasional student from either medicine, nursing, or social
work. To enable maximum nurse participation, meetings are held
when patients are involved in little leaderless sessions. It is important to have all staff present since it is at these meetings that the
bulk of individualized treatment planning is accomplished. In
order to do this the initial task is to collect information from all
of the staff. The supervisor ensures that the psychiatric resident
provides psychological and medical data derived from the patient,
a social worker presents information garnered from the family,
and the nursing staff describes the patient's in-hospital behavior.
After collecting this information the team explores areas of inconsistency between what the patient has said, what the family has
reported, and what has been observed about the patient's behavior. It is important that reports of in-hospital activity be given by
all staff in order to prevent treatment plans from being established that are based on only selected aspects of the patient's
behavior. For example, before proceeding on the assumption that
a patient has, let us say, persistent hyperactivity, it is necessary to
find out if all members of the team have witnessed this kind of
behavior. If not, the team will try to understand why different
people are observing different activities. On the other hand, if the

TABLE IV

TYPICAL PATIENT SCHEDULE ON TOMPKINS-I

MONDAY

8:45 - 9:15 a.m.	Patient-Staff Meeting
9:15 - 10:15 a.m.	Group Therapy
10:30 - 11:45 a.m.	Advisory Board
1:00 - 2:00 p.m.	Gym
2:15 - 3:00 p.m.	Advisory Board
3:00 - 3:30 p.m.	Individual Psychotherapy
5:00 - 5:45 p.m.	Evening Rounds

TUESDAY

9:30 - 10:30 a.m.	Advisory Board
11:00 - 11:45 a.m.	Activities Planning Meeting
1:10 - 2:10 p.m.	Patient-Staff Meeting
2:30 - 3.00 p.m.	Sponsors' Meeting
3:00 - 4:00 p.m.	Little Leaderless
5:00 - 5:45 p.m.	Evening Rounds
8:00 - 9:00 p.m.	Discharge Planning Group

WEDNESDAY

9:00 - 10:30 a.m.	Chief Resident's Rounds
10:30 - 11:30 a.m.	Psychological Testing
1:00 - 1:45 p.m.	Gymnasium
2:00 - 2:45 p.m.	Advisory Board
3:00 - 4:00 p.m.	Big Leaderless
5:00 - 5:45 p.m.	Evening Rounds
7:00 - 8:00 p.m.	Multiple Family Group Therapy

THURSDAY

8:45 - 9:45 a.m.	Group Therapy
10:15 - 11:15 a.m.	Advisory Board
1:00 - 2:00 p.m.	Director's Walking Rounds
3:00 - 4:00 p.m.	Little Leaderless
5:00 - 5:45 p.m.	Evening Rounds

FRIDAY

9:30 - 10:30 a.m.	Patient-Staff Meeting
10:45 - 11:45 a.m.	Advisory Board
1:00 - 2:00 p.m.	Gymnasium
3:00 - 3:30 p.m.	Individual Psychotherapy
5:00 - 5:45 p.m.	Evening Rounds
7:00 - 8:00 p.m.	Evening Activity

SATURDAY

9:30 - 10:30 a.m.	Multiple Family Group Therapy
7:00 - 8:00 p.m.	Evening Activity

SUNDAY

7:00 - 8:00 p.m.	Pass Group

observations are consistent, the team will proceed to the next step which entails the development of an individualized treatment strategy as well as deciding who will be responsible for its implementation.

Although the routine management of patients is executed immediately after the team meeting, major decisions, such as discharge are not implemented until they have obtained the approval of the large staff meeting. These latter meetings include all those who work or train on the unit. They convene three times a week in two hourly sessions and in one thirty-minute meeting. They are conducted by the director or assistant director of the unit and are highly complex administrative and learning experiences. More specifically, their functions are as follows:

1. *Information sharing about current individual patient problems.* Because this is one of its major purposes, the staff meeting begins with the nurses' report of the previous day's activities. The subsequent discussion is focused on serious problems of individual patients.

2. *Discussion about patients not visibly having immediate problems.* It is easy for the T-I as well as any hospital staff to only deal with imminent crises and "forget" about patients who are not presently having any major difficulties. Thus, a systematic attempt is made to periodically discuss these patients. For example, a cooperative patient who has failed to advance on the ladder system for an inordinate period of time will be brought up for discussion.

3. *Presentation of new patients.* The history of all newly admitted patients is briefly presented by a staff member, followed by a short discussion of his tentative treatment plans.

4. *Teaching.* This includes a discussion of a myriad of issues, such as the use of psychoactive medication, family and individual dynamics, and the effective utilization of the unit's complex structure.

5. *Discussion of unit-wide issues and problems.* This refers to the evaluation and resolution of community malfunctions. For

example, if clique formation is excluding certain patients, the staff will decide upon a method of contending with this problem. Other frequently discussed problems are patient secret-keeping, staff dissension, and inadequate performance by the advisory board.

In summary Tompkins-I is an example of a reactive hospital environment that embodies the fundamental principles of a therapeutic community. Although these principles are what specifically characterize a therapeutic community, certain aspects of them can be applied to all forms of psychiatric hospitalization.

BASIC PRINCIPLES OF A THERAPEUTIC COMMUNITY

The fundamental principle underlying the operations of a therapeutic community is that patients assume a major role as *change agents*. By this we mean that patients take a major responsibility for:

1. providing emotional support for other patients
2. offering feedback to other patients and their relatives about their behavior
3. partially determining treatment plans for individual patients
4. implementing these treatment plans, and
5. sharing responsibility for these individual treatment plans as well as some of the overall management of the unit.

Thus, a hallmark of the therapeutic community is that patients assume many of the important therapeutic and administrative functions traditionally assigned to hospital personnel (M. Jones 1953). For example, in the numerous group meetings on Tompkins-I, patients are charged with the tasks of not only offering emotional support to other patients, but providing feedback about their behavior as well. The advisory board is a formal vehicle by which patients make significant decisions about themselves and others. Many management functions of the unit are assumed by the advisory board, members of the Monitor Pool, and Buddy System. (see Appendix A) In this manner patients function as staff, thereby "doing" something rather than only receiving something.

By having patients assume these major responsibilities a number of benefits accrue for both the patients and the staff. Patients are afforded the opportunity to exercise and to expand their interpersonal skills and judgment, thereby raising their self-esteem and counteracting regressive tendencies (Tucker 1973). At the same time patients and staff acquire information about the patient's level of social competence and capacity to tolerate stress by observing his ability to function in these various roles. Although of secondary significance, patients who serve in these capacities free an overburdened staff of many routine responsibilities, allowing them to devote themselves to more specialized tasks. It should be noted that the patient's meaningful participation in the overall treatment program of a therapeutic community should *not* be encouraged in order to create a democratic society. For one thing, nobody has ever shown that democracy "cures" mental illness, or even that democracy can exist in a psychiatric hospital. Unlike the staff the patients generally show a greater degree of impaired behavior, live in the hospital, receive the therapy, and pay the bills. Therefore, one cannot create a fully egalitarian society in a hospital. Nevertheless, patients can assume important therapeutic functions within a psychiatric unit.

In order for patients to do so, a therapeutic community must establish a structure that will facilitate patients serving as change agents. While there are many ways of accomplishing this, we believe that at least seven basic conditions need to be met. First, if patients are to really function as change agents, their *hospitalization needs to be of sufficient duration* so that they can acquire the necessary skills to behave therapeutically towards other patients. This takes time; therefore, because of its relatively brief length of stay, a short-term hospital cannot be expected to maximally utilize patients as change agents (Raskin 1971, Herz 1972a).

Second, while a *primary focus on behavior* is essential for any type of reactive hospital environment, it has additional advantages for a unit which desires to have patients serve as change agents. Overt behavior, unlike the unconscious, can be observed by all patients, regardless of their psychological sophistication, and therefore, they can readily comment upon, influence, and attempt to modify it. In order to make decisions about privileges and responsibilities it is easier for a patient government to base its judgments on overt activity, rather than subtle and oftentimes unverifiable psychodynamic formulations.

Third, for patients to act as change agents the staff needs to share *important clinical data* with the patient community. As a result, the traditional rules of confidentiality need to be modified so that information about the patient remains within the patient-staff community, as opposed to being the exclusive possession of the psychiatrist. Our observations concur with those of Maxwell Jones (1965) in that once patients experience the benefits of having significant therapeutic responsibilities, they no longer are concerned that other patients know about their problems.

Fourth, staff must *establish the expectations* that patients are capable of performing meaningful and important responsibilities (Greenley 1973). If patients' discussions are limited to choosing between bingo and basketball, this cannot be accomplished. Even when making significant decisions, what is of primary import is not that patient government reach "the correct" judgment, but that the patients obtain the experience of being responsible for themselves and learning the consequences of their actions (M. Jones 1953, Grant 1971). The staff demonstrates that they have reasonably high expectations of the patients by allowing them to assume tasks traditionally delegated to hospital personnel. For example, on T-I the staff only vetoes a decision of the advisory board if doing otherwise will have extremely deleterious consequences.

Fifth, a therapeutic community encourages patients to function as change agents by mobilizing and exerting *group pressure* in a multiplicity of settings. For example, on T-I, whether it is in the advisory board, patient-staff meetings, the various group therapies, or even informally between meetings, patients are constantly encouraged by everyone on the unit to act as change agents and to behave responsibly. This pressure persists throughout the day, rather than as in many hospitals where its presence occurs sporadically (if at all) at an occasional group or community meeting. By harnessing the beneficial potential of group pressure and making it an essential feature of a therapeutic community, staff can provide a strong inducement for patients to emit adaptive behaviors while they are assuming therapeutic responsibilities.

Sixth, group pressure can be accentuated when the entire patient community acquires a sense of *shared responsibility*. If patients know that to some extent they will be held personally responsible for each other's behaviors, they will develop a greater desire to act as change agents. For example, on Tompkins-I if a patient has taken illegal drugs, he will receive a severe penalty. As is usually the case other patients may know about this in advance (or have hints to that effect) and fail to act appropriately. In this circumstance the entire patient community will be punished by, let us say, suspending the Buddy System. Implicit in this course of action is the belief that what a minority of patients do will adversely affect the entire community. This position sometimes engenders hostility among some patients who feel they are being punished for the inappropriate actions of others. On the other hand, if used judiciously, placing responsibility on the entire community usually mobilizes group pressure on the individuals involved and accentuates the effect that a patient's anti-social behavior has on the lives of others, in much the same way that it does so in the rest of society.

And finally, a *system of rewards and punishments* should be an integral part of a therapeutic community in order to guarantee that patients will function as change agents. By providing reinforcements, such as the ladder system on T-I, one can boost the patient's motivation to assume responsibility. To a large extent staff expectations, shared responsibility, group pressure, etc. are effective because of the unit's built-in method of providing rewards and punishments via the ladder system.

Bridging the Two Cultures

It is a common phenomenon in psychiatric hospitals to observe the formation of two cultures—one belonging to the patients which operates independently of and at times even antagonistically toward the other belonging to the staff (Stanton 1954, Caudill 1958, Goffman 1961, Ludwig 1966). A way of bridging these cultures is to have patients assume the role of change agents. When this occurs both patients and staff are striving toward the rehabilitation of patient behavior. We are not suggesting that patients and staff share identical values and objectives, but only that the rehabilitation of patient behavior can serve as a common bond between the two cultures.

Insofar as patients assume therapeutic responsibilities for one another, they must establish a value system that is consistent with and conducive to their acting as change agents. On Tompkins-I psychodynamically oriented investigators not affiliated with the unit discovered that the following set of six values[1] pervaded the patient sector (Almond 1968):

1. *Be a member*—be an active member of the T-I system; do not become socially isolated.

2. *Be open*—discuss problems openly with staff and patients; confidentiality is reserved for only the most embarrassing details, such as "being raped by father at age six."

3. *Take responsibility*—by helping others, one helps oneself. Do not rely on others to facilitate magical solutions to your problems.

4. *Have faith in the unit*—believe in the efficacy of T-I and the staff's willingness to be of help.

5. *View family realistically*—recognize the existence of problems within the family and attempt to contend with them realistically.

6. *Face problems directly*—symptoms should not be used as

---

[1] The term *value* is used here to denote ways of thinking, feeling, and behaving on the part of the patients.

"cop-outs" to avoid confronting problems; they should be discussed directly and openly.

These values are never formally prescribed for the patients, but rather were discovered by the investigators to constantly permeate the staff's communications to the patients in a variety of settings, such as individual, group, family, and community meetings. It was found that although different patients subscribed to these values to varying degrees, most of them eventually accepted and actualized them in their daily conduct on the unit. As a result, patients assume a para-staff role and are able to relate to the hospital personnel as respected consultants in a collaborative effort (Almond 1969). It is this collaborative effort, more than anything else, that provides the common bond between the staff and patient culture.

Authority Relationships within a Therapeutic Community

In speaking of a therapeutic community we have deliberately suggested a bridging rather than a fusing of the two cultures. As previously indicated, a psychiatric hospital cannot be an egalitarian order even though patients may play a significant therapeutic role within the unit. Even Maxwell Jones who advocated the democratization of the psychiatric hospital believes that ultimate authority must lie with the staff (Jones 1968). By abdicating this responsibility a unit's program may become an anti-therapeutic experience by floundering into disorganization and possibly chaos (Spadoni 1969, Crabtree 1972). Thus, if a therapeutic community is to be effective, it must be a "guided democracy", with the rights, privileges, and responsibilities of both staff and patients clearly delineated. It is artificial and duplicitous to imply that patients have powers which in reality they do not possess. Conversely, staff should not abridge the tasks and privileges of the patients which by the unit's rules are specifically allotted to patients. For example, on Tompkins-I there often is a temptation on the part of the psychiatrist to bypass the advisory board on any status request and automatically grant it to the patient. Whether this is done for the sake of expediency or in order to "get on the good side of the patient," the net result is that the important role of the advisory board is severely undercut. Thus, patient governments cannot operate effectively unless the staff guarantees that it will be able to utilize its power. In short clearcut authority relationships between patients and staff need to be both clearly established and publicly spelled out.

Although these authority relationships should pervade the totality of staff-patient interactions, it is probably in the large community meetings where they are most distinctly expressed in both word and deed. For instance, on Tompkins-I, the patient-staff meetings are led by a member of the staff who is charged with the responsibility of making the ultimate decisions whether or not to grant a patient's pass request. Although he will attempt to reach a consensus, ultimate authority rests with him. Also, it is his task to structure the meeting around a specific agenda which is mainly provided by the recommendations of the advisory board. Without this type of coherent organization, large community meetings can develop into a highly anxiety producing and confusing experience for many patients, especially those hampered by psychotic thought processes (Herz 1972). We have frequently observed large unstructured meetings dissipate into a kind of "theater of the bizarre" because the actors do not possess any readily accessible mechanisms for transforming chaos into order. Thus, the existence of a structured format provides a clear and concise framework within which patients can be assisted in organizing their thinking and overt behavior.

A more difficult task for the staff of a therapeutic community is to determine which rights, privileges, and responsibilities can and should be delegated to the patients. Although the lack of investigations into this question makes it difficult to reach any definitive conclusions, recently some interesting ideas have been advanced. For example, several authors (Abroms 1971a, Grant 1971) suggest that patients attend staff planning meetings. They argue that patients can provide valuable observations about other patients, help the staff in implementing the treatment program, and learn about themselves and others by listening to the staff's discussion. Abroms (1971a) correctly points out that hospital personnel may be reluctant to admit patients to these meetings because they would have to abandon the use of derogatory remarks and, more legitimately, may be concerned that patients would be unduly upset by the information that would be exchanged. Although the idea of involving patients in staff planning meetings has much to be said for it, especially within a therapeutic community, there are potential difficulties that need serious consideration. For instance, will patient attendance prevent the exchange of critical information, such as "We are presently investigating the possibility that Mr. A. has a brain tumor"? When this was tried in the past on T-I, the meetings readily became perfused with euphemistic terminology and stifled expression of emotionally-laden commentary. Also, it prevented staff from working out their own conflicts over the management of patients.

When attempting to designate which rights, privileges, and responsibilities should be delegated to patients, it is important to remember that such decisions ought to be based solely upon therapeutic rather than ideological considerations. Similarly, this same standard should be utilized when determining the duties of individual staff members. Although hospital personnel ought to expand their repertoire of therapeutic skills, they should not be assigned clinical responsibilities that are beyond their expertise or for which they are not afforded training. Furthermore, within a staff it is important that authority relationships are clearly and openly defined, so that hospital personnel do not exercise authority which in reality they fail to possess. To do otherwise can generate a considerable degree of staff dissension, that ultimately can lead to inferior patient care.

This chapter has limited its discussion to only those major issues that are of special import to a therapeutic community. As one form of psychiatric hospitalization, there are, of course, many other theoretical principles that need to be implemented if a therapeutic community is to become a reactive environment (see chapter 3 and parts III and IV). For now, however, it is important to reemphasize the central principle of a therapeutic community, namely, that patients assume a major role as change agents. The methods enumerated to encourage patients to carry out therapeutic responsibilities emphasize the importance of staff expectations, group pressure, collective responsibility, sharing of clinical information, and the existence of a reward and punishment system. When staff and patients share treatment responsibilities, the rehabilitation of patient behavior can serve as the common link between the frequently existing, and oftentimes antagonistic, two cultures of the psychiatric hospital. And finally, in order that a therapeutic community does not flounder into disarray and disorganization, the necessity of having clearcut and openly expressed authority relationships is stressed. Although instilled with egalitarian sentiments, those who work in a therapeutic community should avoid democratization when it interferes with the rehabilitation of patient behavior.

Chapter 6

THE TOKEN ECONOMY

ONE OF THE MOST RECENT developments in hospital psychiatry has been the emergence of the token economy. The application of behavioral principles, notably those of B. F. Skinner (1938, 1953), generated a wide variety of innovative techniques for the treatment of hospitalized patients (Lindsley 1954, Ayllon 1959) which eventually culminated in the development of the unit-wide token economy system (Ayllon 1965, Schaefer 1969). This unit-wide system was important for many reasons; although they cannot all be mentioned here, a few of them are worth noting. Prior to its development, chronically ill patients would have to be relegated to custodial institutions unless they were among the select few who could afford long-term psychoanalytic facilities. The introduction of the token economy provided a desirable alternative to this undesirable situation. Not only did the emergence of the token economy provide new possibilities for acutely disturbed and chronically ill patients, but also it opened new opportunities for professional mental health workers. Nurses and aides could now play a primary role in active patient care rather than serving as custodians or mere pill pushers and bedpan dispensers. And finally, the token economy system, at least in part, helped psychiatrists focus upon and systematize their thinking about the overt behavior of their patients. Thus, the significance of the token economy cannot be overestimated. Its contribution to hospital psychiatry, although of recent origins, has become increasingly pervasive.

Explicitness, precision, and *accuracy* are the hallmarks of an effective token economy. Each procedure must be specified so that every staff member and patient is fully aware of all details. Thus, patients entering the system may be given a booklet outlining every aspect of the program, and may review it with staff and other more experienced patients (Hersen 1972). Moreover, if the details are not specified accurately, staff will be inconsistent in what they do, and patients, therefore, may flounder in confusion. Vagueness and inconsistency are incompatible with the functioning of the token economy.

Variety is also a crucial ingredient of a successful token economy. There must be a diversity of constructive activities available to patients for which they can receive tokens, as well as an extensive list of ways to exchange them.

Nurses and aides, personnel who are in the most continuous daily contact with the patient, are given major responsibility for running the economy correctly. They determine if a patient has complied with designated criteria so that he may be paid tokens or if he has violated the system and warrants a fine. In order to carry out these tasks effectively, the staff must be fully acquainted with behavioral principles. But this, in and of itself, is insufficient. They must be able to correctly implement the procedures of a token economy by accurately reporting on what they observe and functioning with the utmost of precision and consistency. Thus, staff meetings may be scheduled regularly once or twice each week or even daily, to clarify the operations of the unit and to ensure that the staff is correctly implementing the program.

Candidates for this system are restricted neither by their ages nor by their lengths of stay in the hospital. Token economies have been developed for juveniles (Aitchison 1972) as well as for adults of varying ages.[1] The amount of time a patient spends inside the hospital prior to entering a token economy appears to be not so much a predictor of whether this treatment will work for him but rather a determiner of the kind of aftercare arrangements that are important to plan for him. The long-term patient may require a community based aftercare facility (see Paul 1969). The length of stay variable, however, may partially determine the types of behaviors initially labeled as desirable for him to engage in and the situations—hospital or community—wherein they are performed.

The effects on patients of unit-wide systems differ. For many patients a changeover from a more traditional approach to a token one initiates rebelliousness (Gericke 1965) which, after a time, subsides. Because of their improvement, some patients eventually assume a position in the system where they are responsible, in part, for helping others (Garlington 1966). They may act as controlling influences for other patients by setting standards for them and thereby enhance the successful operation of the token program. The ways in which patients can be employed in aiding other patients both inside and outside the hospital and the many benefits accruing from these efforts to all those concerned warrant further clinical research.

At this point it must be stated that some patients do not seem to benefit from a unit-wide system. For many of these persons *individual* behavioral programs tailored to their specific difficulties may be a more effective alternative (Kazdin 1972a). Techniques pertinent to these programs (e.g., shaping) are outlined in Tables V and VI and discussed in chapter 9.

This chapter, however, will mainly examine the token econ-

---

[1] Because many of the early token economy systems were developed on wards with chronic psychiatric patients, professionals often equate token economy treatment programs as being serviceable only for chronic patients. Furthermore, in addition to token economies in psychiatric hospitals, there currently exist programs in public school classrooms, institutions for the retarded, the home, and other situations.

omy system as it applies to the total structure of a psychiatric hospital unit. In doing so we will first present some illustrations of token economies, and then proceed to discuss basic techniques and principles central to their operation.

SOME EXAMPLES OF TOKEN SYSTEMS

The following report (Lloyd 1970) describes the first 27 months of a long-term token economic system that was designed and implemented in a state hospital for both male and female chronic patients; their median amount of time spent in the institution was 18 years and their median age was 53. Focal behavior areas were grooming and work. Thus, tokens were given for such events as hair combing, being dressed neatly, maintaining schedules, and occupational and industrial activity. (Ten tokens were administered for each hour of work.) Although the above events constituted the main areas dealt with, carrying on appropriate conversations and other desirable social acts as well as taking medications also were rewarded with tokens.

Payments occurred at scheduled times, three per day (7 a.m., 11 a.m., and 4 p.m.), dependent on a patient's earlier performance of a designated positive behavior. For example, patients who had eaten breakfast without undue disruption and sloppiness were paid at the late-morning salary exchange. Eating in a socially appropriate manner comprised: "(1) eating quietly, not gulping food and spending at least 15 min. in the dining hall, (2) tray tidy at the end of meal, and (3) clothing and face not soiled..." (Lloyd 1970) Each one of these activities earned five tokens, making the entire breakfast routine worth 15 tokens. Basic grooming behaviors (e.g., shaving, wearing make-up) were rewarded at the 7 a.m. pay period and working was reinforced in the afternoon.

The reinforceable activities and their payoffs were detailed. But the number of tokens administered depended on the occurrence of a positive behavior and, therefore, could be reduced from the specified amount. This could occur provided the patient did not carry out the behavior properly. For instance according to the authors, if teeth brushing resulted in five tokens, a patient who neglected to use toothpaste would receive only *partial* payment. The system was designed so that token earnings functioned as a barometer of the patient's progress. In general a patient who earned more tokens was doing things more adaptively than his counterpart who earned less.

The most intriguing aspect of this token system was its graduated approach. Those patients who were functioning best were elevated to a position of independence that was off the economy. More specifically, patients could occupy one of three groups, each demanding increased responsibility for self-directed functioning; successful performance in one group brought the patient closer to admission to the next higher level. Under the staff's most stringent control were patients who constituted group one. They spent the majority of their time on the unit. These patients exhibited the most behavioral deficits and maladaptive excesses and were unable to leave the unit except for a short period of work (an hour at a time), for dining, and for some particular recreational activities. In contrast group two patients were allowed more independence. They were permitted home visits and had more possible contacts with the outside community, but lived, albeit in private rooms, on the unit. Unlike the former two groups the last one was entirely removed from the token economy system. They composed a predischarge class of patients demonstrating the most adaptive behaviors, living in another part of the hospital (not in a token unit), and occupying an employee role at the institution.

Criteria for transition from one group to another centered around token acquisition, which reflected the exhibition of increasingly desirable behavior. To advance from the lowest to the middle level required earning 2000 tokens within three weeks. To rise from the middle to the highest status necessitated 10,000 tokens earned by the end of 11 weeks. Demotions occurred as well. For example, if a patient in group three failed to make posthospital plans, he could be returned to group one. Similarly, a middle group patient who was allowed a moderately independent status could be demoted if he did not maintain an earning capacity of at least 200 tokens per week for two weeks in a row.

Therefore, tokens earned, not necessarily saved, was the major variable. Expenditures, of course, took place. Patients spent their tokens on food, living quarters, recreational events, and commodities, such as cigarettes. The greater privileges of increasing one's status also could have been a potent reward for some patients.

The next report (Hersen 1972), in contrast to the one above, deals with relatively young (18-35 years old) veterans, who were admitted for a variety of problems and who stayed in the hospital less than 30 days. Approximately one half of these patients had never before been admitted to a psychiatric hospital.

Target behaviors deemed important to strengthen were in the areas of work, hygiene, responsibility, and occupational therapy, Points were administered to patients when they performed these behaviors. Thus, a patient could earn one point for taking medications on time and five points contingent on two hours of work in the canteen, laundry, laboratory, and so forth. Work assignments were off the unit and were supervised by hospital employees. As the authors note, these supervisors were probably similar behaviorally to typical employers that patients would eventually encounter on the outside.

Generally token economic procedures were operative during the 9 a.m.-5 p.m. day, although fines could be given during the evening for such acts as wearing hospital clothes during non-sanctioned times. Patients could spend their tokens on privileges, the costs being determined by having the residents of the economy rank them on a scale of desirability; prior to the onset of the token program patients were given questionnaires concerning various rewarding activities to find out their preferences. Thus, the opportunities to go on a weekend pass (20 points) or to spend time off the unit participating in recreational activities were earned. During the evening hours, however, most within-hospital activities were administered freely; no token prices were attached to them.

Procedures on the unit were specified clearly so that each incoming patient knew precisely how he could earn and spend his tokens. Daily records of point transactions and weekly patient-staff meetings helped make explicit for everyone all the activities of the token program.

An important feature of this token system was the emphasis placed on *daily planning*. Thus, all members of the unit were instructed to map out exactly what they would be doing for that day including work responsibilities and other activities. The authors noted that this planning requirement seemed to generalize. As a result, patients appeared to be better equipped in thinking through such problems as how they might earn a living once released and how they could effect a better adjustment in the outside community.

The originators of this token economy attempted to evaluate the effects of various procedural changes. The impact of the token approach, *per se*, was determined by gathering data on the patients' behaviors before the program was begun, during it, and when it was temporarily removed. Other variables in addition to the presence or absence of the token system, such as arbitrarily increasing the costs of privileges or giving monetary bonuses also, were judged in terms of their impact on the frequencies of the patients' behaviors. Overall, the results indicated that token economy procedures led to twice the number of adaptive patient behaviors in comparison to no token system. As the authors suggest, the low rate of patient activity in the absence of the token economy resembled the inactivity typically found with chronic patients. In other words when token economic procedures were inoperative, the young more acutely disturbed residents mirrored behaviorally the idleness of long-term non-functioning patients. Can token methods help forestall the growth of these unwanted characteristics? If so, their employment appears to be imperative; certainly, this question is researchable.

Aligned with efforts to discourage the development of chronicity are attempts to strengthen social interactional skills. In this regard Henderson and Scoles (1970) demonstrated the positive effects of token reinforcers on social behaviors. Patients in this token economy were provided with many opportunities (6 nights and 3 days per week) to learn to interact both with other patients and with citizens of the outside community. Such activities as discussion groups, dances, field trips, etc., were made available. A system was devised whereby progressively more reinforcement accrued to patients for performing behaviors that demonstrated greater involvement in the social sphere. The goal was to strengthen behaviors essential to community adjustment. As the authors stated, "Residents engaging in interactions with community persons are paid bonuses in order to foster transition of the resident into the community."

Other token economies have dealt with behaviors similar to those mentioned in the previous reports. More detailed illustrations useful in designing and implementing token systems are provided in Ayllon and Azrin (1968) and Schaefer and Martin (1969). In the remainder of this chapter we will discuss the major characteristics of the token economy alluded to above and some of its underlying principles.

TERMS AND MEANINGS

Every discipline has its own language. Token economy practices represent no exception. The key concept in these programs is *behavior*, but behavior cannot be meaningfully considered in isolation from the environment giving rise to it and sustaining it. Consequently, the patient's activities are viewed in terms of both the situations in which they take place and the effects they produce in the environment. A behavioral description (see Skinner 1969) for any one patient, therefore, basically has three important elements: (a) the *antecedents* to his behavior (i.e., the behavior of others); (b) the *behavior* itself (i.e., the overt activity of the patient); (c) the *consequences* of his behavior (i.e., the critical events that follow it).

Let us briefly consider behavior first. Before any attempt is made to alter the patient's activity, it is important to accurately *define* it. Specific definitions of behavior are a necessary prerequisite to the development of an effective behavior change program. A precise behavioral statement is one in which the relevant characteristics of the activity, in particular those distinguishing it from other activities, are designated. For example, if nurses report that patient A attacks other patients, the exact constituents of this aggression need to be delineated into, let us say, hitting, kicking, or spitting. Also, hitting must be distinguished from touching, etc. The criteria associated with saying that the patient hits someone else must be formally stated so that ambiguity in staff's observing it is reduced. For example, hitting might be defined as "the patient lifting his arm above his head or extending it away from the side of his body and then swinging it towards and making contact with another person." Similarly spitting needs to be distinguished from drooling, and kicking from other movements of the leg. Accurately defined behaviors result in a list of activities that all hospital personnel understand clearly. So defined, these activities are *target behaviors* of an intervention program that is designed to alter them.

Thus, the term "target behavior" emphasizes the attempt made to remove surplus or otherwise confusing meanings from the activity that is dealt with. Suppose, for instance, that you wished to develop neatness in patients. What constitutes being neat? Combing hair, cleaning fingernails, pressing clothes, and so forth are target behaviors that make up the general description, being neat; these activities can be dealt with in the behavioral program. Note that these targets may also require further definition, such as what constitutes clean fingernails.

Another important aspect of behavior concerns the direction in which you want to change it and relatedly how you are going to describe that change. *Direction of change* means strengthening or weakening while *describing that change* entails tabulating its frequency. To strengthen a particular activity (target behavior) means to increase its frequency, that is, to enhance its probability of occurring again in the future, given the right situations. Conversely, to weaken it means to decrease its frequency. Thus, you may want to strengthen a patient's speaking coherently and weaken his delusional statements. You can measure change by counting the number of times each statement occurs in specified situations. Frequency of behavior, however, is not the only way to describe it (c.f., duration, intensity). But it is one of the most valuable ones and, therefore, will be employed in the rest of this chapter except where indicated.

Antecedents and consequences are the influential factors in the present environment of the patient that affect his behaviors. For token economists the major *consequences* of adaptive behavior are called *positive reinforcers*. A positive reinforcer is an event that follows behavior and serves to increase the likelihood that in the future under similar conditions the patient will perform the desired act. For example, if a patient is given cigarettes when he talks coherently, and the number of times he speaks coherently increases, then cigarettes must be acting as positive reinforcers for him. Proof that an event can function as a positive reinforcer for any patient requires that its effectiveness in changing the frequency of his behavior be demonstrated empirically (Skinner 1953).

A positive reinforcer represents only one kind of reinforcer. Another type, *negative reinforcer,* also may be employed to strengthen behavior. This requires some explaining. A negative reinforcer may be thought of as an unpleasant circumstance such as having cold hands, pain, and so forth. Any *activity* that *removes* these hurtful situations or that *avoids* them will be strong. Thus, the behavior of putting on warm gloves when it is chilly, prevents cold hands. Consequently, when it is ten degrees below zero, you will be likely to wear gloves if you are going outside. Note that only when a behavior can be shown to increase in frequency because it postpones or terminates some event, can this event be called a negative reinforcer; thus, establishing that a circumstance is a negative reinforcer must be also demonstrated empirically. Many of life's burdens such as the pain of the dentist's drill or the wrath of a spouse may be viewed as negative reinforcers if they act to increase the frequency of behavior (e.g., dental hygiene practices or fulfilling connubial duties) that enables the individual to escape from these problems or prevent them from arising. Negative reinforcement, that is increasing behavior by having it terminate or postpone distasteful events, is infrequently employed in the token economy, although reports of its use can be found (Cotter 1967). Positive reinforcement, in contrast, is the most often used procedure in token economies and it as well as other techniques will be explained later in this discussion.

Turning now to an examination of the antecedents of behavior, one should note the work of Ivan Petrovich Pavlov. This Russian scientist brought forth numerous links that exist and can be made to exist between one class of behavior, namely, respondents and the stimuli preceding them. The relationships he illuminated are described by the process of classical conditioning (Reynolds 1968, LeBow 1973). The connection between the antecedent stimulus and subsequent response was primary in explaining the occurrence of the behavior—the antecedent stimulus had to be present in order for the behavior, known as a respondent, to take place. Most importantly, the consequences of the respondent behavior in the environment did not enter into altering that stimulus-response relationship. Thus, extending your leg when your knee is tapped is an invariable reflex that an arbitrarily imposed consequence such as five dollars will in no way affect. In this context the leg jerk is a respondent whose occurrence is determined completely by antecedent stimulation, not by what follows it.

Stimuli preceding another class of behavior, known as *operants,* are given greater weight in the design and operation of a token economy. These stimuli become determiners of operant behaviors because of what transpires after operants take place. To more fully understand this statement let us briefly discuss what operant behaviors are. Operants, in contrast to respondents, are activities that are greatly affected by consequences from the environment. What takes place after the operant occurs can alter its strength. Positive reinforcement is an effective procedure for increasing the strength of operant behaviors. That operants can be affected in this way is a fact that is essential to the running of a token economy. This statement means that one task of the hospital staff is to purposely arrange the patient's environment so that his desirable operants such as combing hair, working, speaking coherently, etc., result in positively reinforcing consequences.

Antecedents to operant behaviors control their occurrence because these stimuli have been occasions on which the behaviors have been followed by potent consequences. For example, the presence of an aide (antecedent) may be an occasion that reliably precedes the patient's saying "Hello" (operant) which is followed by a return greeting and perhaps some tokens (consequence). When the patient sees the aide, he greets him and is positively reinforced. We may say that the presence of the aide in the patient's visual field is an effective antecedent to his subsequent behavior *because this subsequent greeting is reinforced*. If positive consequences no longer followed the salutation, the latter probably would decrease and the antecedent controlling it would lose its influence—the "hello" would not occur when the patient saw the aide. A patient in a token economy is confronted by many situations, such as instructions and demonstrations by staff and by other patients, that eventually become important precursors of his operant behavior.

Related to the above discussion are two processes that are important to understand; they are involved in and account for the results of many of the patient's interactions, both planned and unplanned by staff. These processes are *discrimination* and *generalization*. In line with the example just noted, suppose a patient encounters, on an almost daily basis, two other patients—Mr. A and Mr. B—who greet him in the morning with, "Hello, how are you?" You observe that when Mr. A greets the patient, a convivial exchange takes place. But when Mr. B greets the patient, no conversation ensues because the patient ignores him. Our patient responds differently to the other two patients; it may be said that he discriminates between them. To account for this difference in behavior let us say that in the past when Mr. A greeted the patient a cordial interchange ensued. On the other hand when Mr. B greeted the patient and the patient returned the greeting, Mr. B began to vilify him.

Thus, our patient was likely to be rewarded for responding to Mr. A's greeting but not for responding to Mr. B's "Hello." *Different consequences followed our patient's salutatory behavior in the presence of the two other patients.* Consequently, he learned to respond *differentially* to them. In the presence of one individual our patient's response was cordial, but in the presence of the other one, it was not. The example illustrates the process of discrimination. Complex and subtle discriminations reflect the activities of everyone who successfully adjusts to living in the natural environment. Such events as the tone of a friend's voice, the look in a loved one's eyes, various activities of a boss, traffic signs along the road, etc., are all antecedent stimuli that control different behaviors leading to various results. In fact it may well be his difficulty in recognizing and discriminating between subtle cues that often leads to an individual's being seen as maladaptive.

Generalization, behaving similarly in a variety of situations, describes a process that is the converse of discrimination. The patient who discriminates behaves differently in similar situations (following similar antecedents). But the patient who generalizes behaves similarly in a wide variety of situations. The terms overgeneralization and overdiscrimination illuminate the continuous nature of the two processes and highlight their potentially negative extremes.

The generalization of positive activities that originate in the hospital must continue to occur in other environments following discharge if rehospitalization is to be avoided. Techniques useful in fostering the generalization of behavior change may be found elsewhere in the literature on behavior modification (Bandura

1969, Franks 1969, LeBow 1973). Broadly speaking, for the psychiatric patient, generalization and discrimination are both processes central to effective readjustment.

Another term frequently found in token economy reports is *contingency*. It describes the relationship between behavior and some event subsequent to its occurrence, such as the presentation of a positive reinforcer, the removal of a negative reinforcer, and others. Some basic contingencies useful in token economy programs will be examined later. If the token program is to realize any positive effect, contingencies must be planned, not left to accident. Thus, to strengthen adaptive behavior in a psychiatric unit, staff must purposely arrange the patient's environment to systematically react to his desirable behavior—the patient's behavior must *produce* positive reinforcers; when this is accomplished positive reinforcers can be said to be contingent on his behavior. If the target behavior occurs, the reinforcer is administered. That positive reinforcers (e.g., tokens) must be contingent on appropriate behavior in order for it to be strengthened is a major operational principle of a token economy. To become frequent, behavior must pay off.

OBSERVING AND RECORDING PATIENTS' BEHAVIORS

Keep accurate data. This is a basic rule for operating an effective token unit. One unique feature of the psychiatric hospital in contrast to the outside environment is that comprehensive data collection is made possible, because patients are under the aegis of the staff on a near 24-hour basis. As soon as the patient enters the unit, complete recording of his activities may begin. Then nurses and aides can chart what he does and record all token transactions with which he is involved during the entire period of his hospitalization.

To precisely record behavior one must define it. At least two recorders should be able to agree on what they observe. In token economic systems, desired behaviors are comprehensively listed along with their earning power. The objective is that the patient explicitly understand all the contingencies. For the same reason, positive reinforcers such as cigarettes, passes, etc., are clearly specified in conjunction with their costs in tokens. A wide variety of behaviors and positive reinforcers is sought in order to maximize the suitability for the patient of the activities he engages in and to motivate his performance. With a large number of alternatives, not a small amount, the patient has greater latitude in his choices.

Various behaviors can be labeled as desirable by staff and hence remuneratory. Thus, activities relating to work, self-care, responsibility, social interaction, and self-control can be targets (Carlson 1972, Kazdin 1972b). The major criterion for choosing to classify an activity as a target behavior should be its total relevance to the patient's well-being; this involves its meaningfulness to him and to society (cf. Baer 1968, Ayllon 1972, LeBow 1973). Lists of reinforceable and punishable activities (e.g., unit-rule violations) can be drawn up for all patients demonstrating particular problems.

Finding positive reinforcers is possible by simply observing what patients do often. Ayllon and Azrin (1965) effectively incorporated this principle into the development of their token economy program. From the basic work of Premack (1959, 1963), one can accurately conclude that numerous reinforcers, which may be used to strengthen various behaviors, are available. Generally, Premack showed that a behavior which is frequently emitted—a behavior of high probability—can be employed to strengthen a behavior of lower probability. In the psychiatric hospital this finding means that the opportunity to go on a pass, the opportunity to sit in a room, the opportunity to go to a movie, etc.—*whatever the patient seems to want to do as evidenced by what he does when given the chance*—may be employed to facilitate the occurrence of desired activities such as social interaction, going to the dining room and eating, talking to nurses, and so forth—*whatever seems important for the patient to do more often*. Before beginning the operation of a token unit, Hersen (1972) assigned costs to reinforcing activities on the basis of the patients' labeling these events as attractive; a questionnaire was given to assess the patients' views on this subject.

When tokens are administered or taken away, one should endeavor to list all persons involved in each transaction (e.g., staff and patients). In addition one should write down the behavior involved as well as the amount of tokens exchanged. Once again, complete data must be kept.

Inclusive records are essential for several reasons. First they help the staff decide what alterations in the program are necessary to ensure its continuing to work in the patient's best interests. For example, if a patient is hoarding tokens, specific strategies may need to be developed for him, or some change in available back-up reinforcers (e.g., cigarettes, passes, etc.) may be necessary. The main point is that information regarding the activities of the patient constitutes feedback for the staff to revise, as seems appropriate, the contingencies in operation. This corrective feature of a behavior modification program is summarized by the following dictum: "Let the patient's behavior be your guide." Accurate monitoring of the patient's activities is a requirement of a well designed token system. Another reason for having comprehensive behavioral records has to do with *maintaining accuracy*. Reliable observation of the patient's behaviors is a vital aspect of any behavior modification program (see S. M. Johnson 1973). Various staff activities in relation to patients' behaviors also need to be defined and observed. For example, an important activity of staff is giving patients tokens contingent on appropriate behavior. Direct observation of staff by other staff is periodically necessary to ascertain if token administration is occurring according to the criteria set up (see Ayllon 1968).

A third reason for stressing that complete records are vital reiterates, in part, our previous discussions of clearly defining target behaviors and tabulating their frequency. Simply stated, comprehensive behavioral records help staff *formulate objectives for individual patients and devise meaningful intervention plans for them.* Without such data, designing workable techniques for specific patients on the token unit is hampered.

Fourth, behavioral records *provide basic evaluative information.* These types of data are necessary in dealing with specific patients with "special" difficulties refractory to the general unit-wide system, and in ascertaining the effectiveness of the token procedures for the entire ward. With regard to the latter Hersen (1972) showed the utility of gathering data prior to the implementation of the token methods in order to help determine if they were *the* effective variables responsible for altering the patients' behaviors; this first stage is called pre-treatment or baseline assessment. In the Hersen study it generated the standard for drawing conclusions about the significance of the token system. Pre-treatment to treatment contrasts, however, do not represent the complete evaluative design that may be used to measure the importance of the token procedures for the entire unit or for individual patients *per se* (see chapter 15).

The task of evaluating procedures is not only important for patients who are currently members of the token system, but also for those individuals yet to be a part of it. Evaluative data obtained through careful observation allows staff to determine whether token economic procedures are functionally related to any positive behavior changes that have ensued for all patients considered as a group or for specific patients undergoing more tailored programs. In addition, by *repeatedly evaluating* what they are doing for current patients, staff achieve a better understanding of the methods at their disposal. This greater knowledge of behavioral technology should affect their sophistication in choosing potentially effective procedure for future patients.

Finally, detailed behavioral records taken during the patient's stay in the hospital are a *major component to any follow-up measures* of his progress. Both the durability and the generalization of his desirable behavior change in the outside environment need to be assessed if a judgment is to be made that the token system had an extensive effect on him. Sadly, the majority of available evidence reflects the dearth of empirically based claims for long-term results (Paul 1969, Agras 1972b, Carlson 1972) but the basic technology for affecting post-hospital functioning is available and may be developed further by applying behavioral techniques in the patient's post-hospital environment (Paul 1969, Kazdin 1972b, see chapter 14). Detailed follow-up assessment data will quite obviously serve as the foundation for future statements about the long-term efficacy of token economic systems in the psychiatric hospital.

A variety of methods exists for obtaining precise records of behavior and the conditions where it takes place (Hall 1970, LeBow 1973). For example, behaviors can be tallied each time they occur in a specified situation (i.e., event recording) or they can be observed for their occurrence or non-occurrence in selected small intervals of time. Observations could be taken, let's say, in two-minute intervals for 30 minutes, three times per day, making a total of 45 two-minute intervals of observation time; this is *interval recording*.

A recording technique that is particularly well suited to the operation of a psychiatric unit is called *time-sampling* (Ayllon 1963). It allows for recording, with a minimum amount of effort, a large number of patient behaviors that occur in specific contexts. Schaefer and Martin (1966), for example, report a study in which systematic observations were collected, using time-sampling, on 40 patients all of whom were members of a token economy unit. Whether a patient emitted one or more than one behavior at the time he was observed was found to be related to his being judged as apathetic. More specifically, those patients who generally were noted to be *only* "walking", "running", "standing", "sitting", or "lying down" were labeled as more apathetic than patients usually found to be engaged in a greater variety of activities. To gather precise assessments of apathy, staff constructed checklists detailing various behaviors; for ease of record keeping, activities were coded with a number. According to the authors, the five behaviors mentioned above, no two of which could occur at the same time, were listed. In addition other activities that could take place when the five mutually exclusive ones occurred were catalogued. Time-sampling happened in the following ways: once each half-hour, thirty times per day for several days, staff observed and recorded the patient's single and combined activities. Only a few seconds of staff time were needed to complete any one period of observation. From the accumulated behavioral data, an apathy rating for each patient could be determined and utilized in his treatment plan.

TOKENS: WHAT THEY ARE AND WHY THEY ARE EMPLOYED

Tokens are concrete objects that can be used as positive reinforcers in a token economy. Such things as metal objects that have been specially marked, foreign coins of low monetary value, paper that functions as money, different color poker chips, and so forth may serve as tokens. It is necessary that whatever is employed be hard to counterfeit, simple to administer, and easy to carry by staff and patients alike (see Ayllon 1968). Recently, many token economists have switched from the use of a physical token to points or other circumscribed yet less tangible units for rewarding behavior. For example, Aitchison (1972) described an inexpensive system for giving points rather than the more customary tokens in a situation where there was a ratio of 50 patients to five aides. Although tokens may take longer to administer and are more cumbersome than points, they may serve as more concrete measures of the effects of behavior. Thus, the token is a tangible representation of what the individual has accomplished and may accentuate the contingency between the activity and its consequence (Skinner 1953).

Regardless of which approach is used, however, either points or tokens can function as vehicles for strengthening desirable patient behavior. Tokens, etc., *per se* have no positive value, in and of themselves. Tokens or points, like money, gain their potency as reinforcers by being essential in acquiring other positive consequences. In other words when the patient possesses tokens he can purchase a variety of things that he wants, such as better living accommodations, tobacco, the opportunity to leave the unit for the weekend, or even to buy his way out of the token system (e.g., Atthowe 1968). It is the various things that tokens will purchase that provide them with their value.

But simply giving the patient tokens is insufficient. Tokens must be given on contingency, that is they must be administered because specified behaviors have occurred. It is the contingency between behavior and the potent consequences that is crucial. That reinforcers should be contingent on behavior simply defines one rule of their proper administration.

Another aspect of appropriately giving tokens is concerned with their immediacy. For most patients in a psychiatric unit *immediate reinforcement* is important. A long delay between the patient's behaving in a desired way and his receipt of tokens may retard his progress. For others, especially those who are further advanced, a delay may not be so detrimental and may even be worthwhile. For instance, deferred payment for working is customary in society. In this regard Atthowe and Krasner (1968) developed a successful token economy program for psychiatric patients where some of them—the ones who had made noticeable progress—were paid on a weekly basis rather than immediately for engaging in specific work behaviors.

But immediacy of token reinforcement may be most essential in the beginning stages of the patient's treatment. Problems exist, however, in arranging the environment so that reinforcers other than tokens can be given promptly after a designated activity occurs. Going on a pass, for example, would be almost impossible to administer immediately—the patient cannot be released from the hospital each time he does something worthwhile. Similarly, other positive reinforcers, such as going to a movie, simply cannot be given for every appropriate behavior. Not only would the patient soon lose interest in them, resulting in a loss of their effectiveness, but also his continual removal from the treatment program would inordinately delay, if not prohibit, his progress. Reinforcers such as cigarettes, etc., however, might be administered immediately provided that the patient could be persuaded not to consume them right away and thereby not to take time away from the desirable activity. But even with these rewards, problems exist. For one thing if these consequences were employed frequently, the risk of early satiation would be great. For practicality, convenience, and effectiveness, therefore, the range of non-token reinforcers that could be employed in a psychiatric unit and delivered immediately would be small and would require constant variation. Many patients might be unmotivated by these rewards and consequently would be unlikely to engage in the activities that produced them. And, thus, effective behavioral treatment would be hampered.

The token is the way out of these problems. First, patients do not tire of receiving them—satiation is improbable. Second, they may be administered promptly without necessarily leading to the removal of the patient from the therapeutic situation in which his desirable behaviors are occurring. Third, they create access to a very wide range of rewards. Simply stated, the patient can learn to save his tokens in order to buy a pass, or time watching T.V., etc. Because these positive reinforcers are now available to him, he will be induced to perform the adaptive activities that staff have listed. Thus, the token is of value as an *intermediary* between the desired behavior and the desired positive reinforcer (back-up reinforcer); because of this position the token itself becomes a reinforcer that can be given immediately without inordinately delaying treatment or without rapidly producing satiation.

In addition to being a medium of exchange the token is also functional in helping the patient become more responsive to other, more naturally occurring reinforcers, such as praise and attention. Because these latter reinforcers are customarily employed by the outside community, his sensitivity to them is important for sustaining his post-hospital adjustment. Simply stated, the token may be used in aiding the patient's coming into contact with social reinforcers. This is possible by juxtaposing social consequences with tokens and gradually discontinuing the tokens while maintaining approval, etc. For instance, in the early phases of the behavioral program, each time the patient engages in the behavior he should be immediately given approval and a token, in that order. Then, gradually, the administration of tokens should be reduced subsequent to each occurrence of the behavior, as the social reinforcer (e.g., approval) becomes more powerful. For many patients, responsiveness to social reinforcers is already there but for others it is not. More tragically, for many patients who are initially responsive to these important events, long-term non-reactive hospitalization can act to retard this sensitivity.

In addition to social reinforcers the kinds of positive consequences that a patient may be helped to come into contact with via the token may be those related to his own progress. This is suggested by the following example. Leitenberg, Agras, and Thomson (1968) reported a study in which a hospitalized anorexic female was helped initially through a systematic program of social and material rewards administered contingent on her exhibiting adequate levels of eating. The removal of extrinsic incentives, however, did not result in the predicted decrement in this desirable behavior. The authors postulated that the noticeable improvements that the patient herself *eventually* was able to visualize emanating from her increased food consumption could have become the most powerful reward in the program. If so, taking away extrinsic incentives would not alter her eating behaviors. Thus, the patient's beneficial eating responses, at some point, could have generated rewards that made the use of externally imposed maintaining events, such as "privileges," unnecessary. Perhaps, as the authors conjectured, external rewards may serve to tangibly confirm for the patient the progress he eventually notes and after awhile may become trivial in sustaining his adaptive efforts.

The critical consequences of the patient's behaviors are those affecting his long-term functioning (e.g., Ferster 1967). In a token economy when the most powerful consequences of relevant conversation is feedback from others, which is instrumental in acquiring many additional rewards, the individual will be more likely to evidence an extended verbal repertoire than when the consequence of his speaking coherently is only a token backed up by food, cigarettes, etc. But as suggested, these material events (e.g., food) may be imperative in first bringing the patient into contact with the more naturally available rewards (Bandura 1969).

TECHNIQUES USED IN THE TOKEN ECONOMY

Positive reinforcement is the most powerful and frequently used technique in the token economy. Its major function, as indicated, is to strengthen behavior. When the patient goes to work and completes the job satisfactorily, for example, he will receive tokens which can be exchanged for various things he wants. Thus, *the positive reinforcement procedure* describes the purposely arranged contingent relationship between specific behaviors and tokens. More colloquially, the patient is given something pleasant for doing something adaptive.

It is evident from what has been said previously that the entire unit-wide structure of the token system is based upon the utility of this procedure for strengthening behavior. The positive reinforcement procedure also is effective, in specifically designed behavior modification programs, for patients who are unresponsive to the global token program or who are given behavioral treatment on a unit not totally run according to the token system (see chapter 9). With regard to the latter, for instance, Smith and Carlin (1972) reported success in helping a 22-year-old female patient control her hysterical crying and tantrums, as well as various postural mannerisms. The patient received points contingent upon her acting appropriately for specified periods of time. Time off the unit was a major back-up reinforcer that points could buy. Soon after the onset of the programs, the patient was discharged from the hospital. The authors found no return of her aberrant behaviors. A sobering comment in the report was that before discharge but after a brief period of success with the program the patient once again began acting in her deviant ways; nevertheless, the point regimen was continued and, within a short time, the patient demonstrated control once more. This "holding tough," at least for a week or so in many cases, is necessary if the behavior modification program eventually is to take effect. Another extremely important aspect of this rehabilitation plan was the emphasis placed on completely specifying procedures that were used as well as behaviors that were reinforced. The nurses and attendants who carried out the program were apprised of all relevant details and this structuring, as the authors point out, may have been instrumental in securing staff's cooperation.

Two procedures for weakening behavior (i.e., reducing its frequency), often cited as being used on the psychiatric unit, are *extinction* and *response-cost*. Extinction is the opposite of positive reinforcement[1]. Whereas the latter involves presenting a pleasant event contingent on behavior, extinction entails the discontinuation of the event. Note that extinction does not depict a contingent relationship between behavior and a consequence, but rather describes a way to break-up the contingency—a particular behavior simply is no longer followed by the positive reinforcer that previously was given subsequent to it. For example, Ayllon and Michael (1959) reduced the disruptive behaviors of a female psychiatric patient by removing the positive reinforcers believed to be maintaining these acts. The patient made continual visits to the nursing station, causing the nurses much harassment. To quell her bothersomeness (and the nurses' ill feeling towards her), the authors implemented an extinction procedure. More specifically, it was reasoned that attention from the nurses, albeit negative, was perpetuating the difficulty—functioning as a positive reinforcer—so removing it should result in a less frequently occurring

---

[1] There are extinction techniques that can be viewed as opposites of the negative reinforcement operation (see Bandura 1969, pp. 385-414).

problem. Therefore, the nurses were instructed to stop cajoling and coaxing the patient out of the office, and instead, were told simply to ignore her when she appeared. In approximately seven weeks the patient's visits decreased to a more tolerable range. Thus, extinction involved the discontinuation of the positive reinforcer that was believed to be maintaining the problem. Its ease of administration and effectiveness make it a worthwhile technique to use in any psychiatric unit (cf. Ayllon 1964).

Response-cost, the second procedure, consists of staff's removing tokens from the patient when he performs undesirable activities. In contrast to extinction this technique describes a contingent relationship between behavior and subsequent events—the occurrence of unwanted behaviors results in the forfeiture of positive reinforcers (tokens). Response-cost is frequently employed in the token economy. Upper (1971), for example, reports removing tokens for patient infractions. This procedure was successful in reducing these undesired activities. The amount of each fine was determined by the staff in advance and was dependent on the felt seriousness of the offense.

Some token economists eschew the merit of response-cost, preferring to minimize all forms of punishment. One way of decreasing undesired behavior without resorting to any type of penalty is to positively reinforce the patient for activities incompatible with the ones to be weakened—*reinforcing other behavior* (see LeBow 1973). For instance, instead of forfeiting tokens for a patient's continual complaining (i.e., response-cost), progressively longer periods of not complaining could be rewarded. Complaining and not complaining are mutually exclusive and strengthening the latter should inhibit the former. Further, a patient who frequently sits in his room may be positively reinforced for going to a work assignment with other people in the hospital. Work and isolation are incompatible. Strengthening adaptive behaviors should, in general, obviate anti-social ones, a view central to the operations of various token systems (see Ayllon 1972).

Other procedures have been incorporated into the operation

of the token system. Some, such as shaping, are relevant to programs specifically designed for individual patients (see Tables V and VI).

TABLE V

INTERVENTION PROCEDURES FOR PRODUCING AND FOR STRENGTHENING BEHAVIOR[1]

Technique	Definition
Positive Reinforcement	Positive Reinforcement is a method for increasing the frequency of a desired behavior by presenting a pleasant event (e.g., offering candy, praise, or money), contingent on the occurrence of the behavior. The staff must arrange the patient's environment so that the desirable behavior produces the positive reinforcer.
Shaping	Shaping is a procedure for producing a behavior in order that the Positive Reinforcement method may be implemented for increasing it. This is to be done by reinforcing the essential components that make up the target behavior so it will take place. The target behavior is produced by providing reinforcement for steps (actions) that move progressively closer to it. For example, to strengthen bathing independently, it is necessary to begin positively reinforcing the patient whenever he initiates a step that is in the direction of this activity (e.g., undressing himself, walking to the shower room unassisted, etc.) . The execution of all the parts results in the desired activity.
Instructing	Describing a behavior to be performed, instructions are stimuli that the staff gives to the patient. They should be clear, should be explicit, and should always specify exactly what behaviors are requested. Performing them should be immediately reinforced. Target behaviors easy for the patient to perform may be described in their entirety. Complex target behaviors difficult for the patient to perform should be broken down into their parts (steps) and should be arranged sequentially. Then each element should be instructed and its performance should be reinforced. Proceeding to a new step should occur when the patient has mastered the preceding ones. Once each of the steps constituting the complex behavior has been learned, all of them may be instructed, and the performance of the entire behavior may be reinforced.

(continued on next page)

TABLE V *(continued)*

INTERVENTION PROCEDURES FOR PRODUCING AND FOR STRENGTHENING BEHAVIOR[1]

Technique	*Definition*
Demonstration-Imitation	Demonstration-Imitation is one procedure that may be used in helping a patient to produce a behavior. By observing the staff clearly demonstrate an activity and by being reinforced for correctly imitating it, a patient can learn a new behavior or can increase the complexity of some other one that he can already perform. If the activity to be produced and then to be accelerated is complex, the following steps are valuable: (a) specify the target behavior, and sequentially arrange the parts which compose it, from first to last; (b) demonstrate each part clearly; (c) reinforce the patient's correct imitation of each element shown; (d) advance from one step to the next only when the patient masters the previous ones. When all the parts can be performed correctly, they may be linked together to form the whole target behavior, which is then demonstrated in its entirety. The imitation of the total target behavior becomes the requirement for reinforcement.
Negative Reinforcement............	Negative Reinforcement is a procedure for increasing the frequency of a desired behavior by removing or by postponing an unpleasant event contingent on the occurrence of the activity. Negative Reinforcement requires that the staff arrange the patient's environment in such a way that the occurrence of a desirable behavior removes or postpones some unpleasant consequence.

[1] Reprinted with modifications from M. D. LeBow, *Behavior Modification: A Significant Method in Nursing Practice,* New Jersey: Prentice-Hall, Inc., 1973.

TABLE VI

Intervention Procedures for Weakening Behavior[1]

Technique	Definition
Aversive Stimulation	Aversive Stimulation is a procedure in which a painful or unpleasant event such as a verbal reprimand, shock, or noise is presented contingent on the occurrence of an undesirable behavior.
Withdrawal of Positive Reinforcement	Withdrawal of Positive Reinforcement is a procedure in which a positive reinforcer is removed, denied, or ended contingent on the occurrence of an undesirable behavior.
(a) Response-Cost	Response-Cost involves the subtraction of positive reinforcers from a pool of available reinforcers contingent on undesirable behavior.
(b) Time-Out	Time-Out involves the temporary removal of the patient from a reinforcing situation contingent on his emitting an undesirable behavior (e.g., he is sequestered for awhile in a room devoid of positive reinforcers).
Reinforcing Other Behavior	Reinforcing Other Behavior is a procedure in which an unwanted activity is decreased by administering positive reinforcers contingent on the occurrence of desirable behavior which is incompatible with the undesirable behavior. An incompatible behavior is any activity that does not occur at the same time as the undesirable behavior.
Extinction	Extinction, as it applies to positively reinforced behavior, is a procedure in which the positive reinforcers that have followed the occurrence of the behavior are discontinued.
Satiation	Satiation is a procedure in which large quantities of a positive reinforcer (usually related to the undesirable behavior) are made available to the patient until the undesirable behavior decreases.

---

[1] Reprinted with modifications from M. D. LeBow, *Behavior Modification: A Significant Method in Nursing Practice*, New Jersey: Prentice-Hall, Inc., 1973.

REINFORCING STAFF PERFORMANCE

In chapter 15 we will examine the manner in which personnel in different types of units (e.g., therapeutic communities, token economies) can be taught to improve their skills. A major aspect of this instruction is related to *maintaining* a high level of staff performance after the teaching program ends. Rephrased, this concern is with finding ways of reinforcing staff for their positive efforts in relation to patients; the goal is that staff will continue interacting with patients beneficially. Unfortunately, that patients get better, as mentioned in chapter 3, may not be the significant factor in motivating staff's continuing efforts.

The literature on reinforcing staff in a behavioral treatment setting is deficient. In one report, however, Panyon, Boozer, and Morris (1970) did describe a procedure of some merit. The authors provided attendants of retarded children in an institutional setting with feedback concerning the number of teaching sessions they conducted with the children, subsequent to the conclusion of a course of training in behavior modification. A feedback sheet denoting the activities of the aides, constructed by the staff psychologist, was presented to the attendants once each week, and then was posted in a highly visible place on the unit. Feedback was effective in getting the attendants to implement their previous teachings. Panyon *et al.* noted that delaying the institution of this procedure inhibited the aides' susceptibility to it. Thus, as the authors suggested, a feedback program should be started soon after formal behavior modification training ends to ensure that attendants begin early to implement and continue to implement their new skills.

In a similar vein Katz, Johnson, and Gelfand (1972) provided extra money for aides in a psychiatric hospital when they increased the number of times they appropriately rewarded specific patients, who beforehand were relatively unaffected by the ongoing token contingencies. Extrinsic reinforcement given to aides for precisely administering frequent reinforcement to patients was an efficient strategy; that is, not only did aides increase their skillfulness, but also patients who were recipients of the positive reinforcers demonstrated more appropriate work-oriented activities. Unhappily, not too long after the money contingency was withdrawn from the aides, their betterment as well as the concomitant gains made by the patients decreased. The temporary nature of the aides' improvement underscores the importance of researching how positive reinforcers can be used to durably modify staffs' behaviors. Money, feedback, bonuses, and vacations are some possible reinforcers (Ayllon 1968, Panyon 1970).

It may be that patient improvement is either a null reinforcer or too delayed (Panyon 1970) to maintain the efforts of many overburdened hospital personnel. A possible solution to this difficulty, suggested by Katz (1972), is to utilize undergraduate college students as part-time helpers on the token economy unit; their major responsibility would be to implement behavior modification practices for the patients.

Psychiatric hospital administrators could harvest many benefits from directly employing or in other ways tapping the supply of potentially available behavioral technicians who exist in the natural environment. A cadre of behavior modification experts could be instrumental in carrying out necessary follow-up evaluations, could implement many aspects of the unit-based token system, and perhaps, most importantly, could provide assistance to patients and their families in developing home-centered programs that would sustain and broaden the progress made by the patient during his hospitalization. The benefits of the token economy could be extended to the outside environment with the help of paraprofessionals who are taught to utilize behavioral practices in that context and who are paid for their services.

This approach or something akin to it is desperately needed if the token economy system is to achieve the goal of long-term extra-hospital adjustment for its patients. In short the post-hospital functioning of the patient must become a major concern of the within hospital system. This concern is not only with nurturing the development inside the unit of behaviors essential for functioning outside of it. Nor is it just with giving the patient experiences that partially mirror what the natural environment provides (e.g., Hersen 1972). But, also it means arranging the patient's post-hospital environment so that it can become more reactive to him.

Thus far, this chapter has attempted to draw together the main ingredients of the token economy. In the last section we will try to elucidate the basic underpinnings of this system.

Behavioral principles underlie the operation of the token economic approach for dealing with human problems. One of the most influential of these has been indicated throughout this chapter, namely that behavior and the environment interact. Behavior affects and in turn is affected by the environment. To change behavior one must change the environment. For the staff of a token economy unit, the implications of this principle are clear: arrange the patient's environment so that his adaptive behavior pays off. Conversely, if you want the patient to stop behaving in deviant ways stop the pay off, provide him with alternative ways of behaving that do pay off (or do both), or fine him. The economic nature of the token system reflects the economic phraseology of these statements.

Another tenet underpinning behavioral treatment in general and token economic systems in particular is that focusing treatment on buried intrapsychic structures is unnecessary for helping patients recover. Rather than seeking to disinter buried internal etiologic psychological conflicts, the token economist attacks the behavior problems directly. Thus, token economists try to program events in the patient's external environment that are or can become functionally related to his adaptive behavior.

Is vs. Does Statements

Token economists, generally, are more concerned with what patients "do" than what they "are." For many more traditional therapists, "is" statements, such as Mr. P "is" passive, "is" lacking in self-esteem, etc., serve as the bases for describing him. In contrast token workers are likely to shun these "is" statements. Simply put, token economists feel that "is" statements are barren, not indicative of what is wrong and, relatedly, not suggestive of potentially effective treatments. "Does" statements, however, such as Mr. A cries in his room at night, hits people, and so forth are more useful. They are usually more closely tied to environmental conditions instrumental to the patient's rehabilitation; "does" statements help to remove the uncertainties from patient description.

Measurable Products

To be useful, a "does" statement must be measurable. Frequency of behavior, as indicated, serves the task of measurement very well, provided that specific definitions of behavior are made. Thus, "is" descriptions first must be translated into what the patient "does"; this is possible through preliminary observations (see Bijou 1968). Then, the resulting "does" statements are broken down into their behavioral constituents. Because we have already examined this notion, we will now concern ourselves with the reliability of behavioral measurement.

Reliability refers to the degree of agreement between two or more observers that a particular patient has or has not behaved in a designated way. The problem we are discussing is one of human measurement. More specifically, do the assessments made by one observer coincide with the assessments made by another observer about what a third person has done? Is the information obtained unbiased by the predilections or vagaries of the measurers?

To the degree that biased observations are minimal the level of agreement among observers will approach 100%. Conversely, if the behaviors have been left undefined or if the observers' expectancies, etc., interfere with their observing, the level of agreement will be low—close to 0%. If behavioral observations are unreliable, carefully selecting intervention procedures and evaluating their effects for any patient will be difficult, if not impossible. Reliable behavioral measurement is essential to the development of a meaningful behavioral program. Techniques for ascertaining the reliability of behavioral observations are available in the behavior modification literature (see Hall 1970, LeBow 1973).

To a large extent, therefore, the emphasis on measurable products highlights the de-emphasis by token economists on attempting to uncover poorly identified intrapsychic mechanisms. Furthermore, the emphasis on reliably measuring behavior partially explains why many token economists prefer to deal with overt rather than covert acts (e.g., ruminative obsessions), although these latter types of behaviors are neither denied importance nor overlooked in the behavior modification literature (e.g., Skinner 1953, Jacobs 1971).

Deprivation

The issue of whether deprivation is an ethical and justifiable tool of the behavior modifier has stirred controversy from many mental health professionals (Ball 1968, Bragg 1968, Cahoon 1968, Lucero 1968, Miron 1968). Polarized opinions for and against its employment have made deprivation a legitimate issue for discussion. In its worst form deprivation means the total denial of basic necessities (food etc.), pleasures, and rights akin to the insufferable regimen that millions of people experienced in concentration camps. For many professionals the term conjures up exactly that sort of meaning and to even consider deprivation as a tool is unconscionable.

To be clearer about what deprivation is when employed by trained persons in the psychiatric unit, let us define it. Simply stated, deprivation is a process that enhances the subsequent use of rewards. In a behavior modification program, for example, the use of food as a reward for some behavior will only be possible if the individual is hungry. Therefore, some period of reduced food intake or abstinence will have to precede using food as a reward—food deprivation. A period of semi-denial prior to its use will make it more effective as a strengthener of behavior.

The effectiveness or potency of a reward is critical to the patient's recovery. That is why strong reinforcers are necessary to programs wherein the positive reinforcement procedure is used. Deprivation as a functional part of the patient's treatment must be judged in terms of its worthiness in helping the patient recover relative to its ill effects when evaluated alone (Cahoon 1968). The question certainly is not whether to use the form of deprivation that was described initially. If extreme forms of deprivation appear to be necessary in order for the reinforcer to become potent, then something is awry with the behavioral program being tried. The question is really whether to employ processes that make rewards more effective in facilitating the occurrence of adaptive behavior. The answer is clear for the token economist—procedures that help programs work *for the patient's best interests* must be used.

In most token economies the notion of deprivation of reinforcers can be translated best into the *controlled use of reinforcers* (Ball 1968). Making available a wide variety of reinforcers, such as weekend pass, the opportunity to go to a dance, etc., that are purchased by the patient with tokens he has earned obviates the necessity of using primary events as major reinforcers. If going on a pass is a potent back-up reinforcer for the patient, it is only necessary to provide him with the opportunity to do so, if he has engaged in enough appropriate behaviors; its administration is not freely given, it is controlled. Severe denial of basic necessities is contraindicated by the operation of the token economy.

Control

Control like its often maligned counterpart, manipulation, may be damned as opposed to the patient's welfare. To say we should not control, however, is tantamount to saying that we should not alter conditions affecting the patient's behavior. And that view would deny treatment in general; in fact it could justify custodialization. The patient's behavior in the psychiatric hospital is affected as much by neglect as it is by the judicious application of positive reinforcement.

Whether we like it or not we do control the patient's behavior in the psychiatric unit and we must recognize this fact. The most sensible concern is how best can the psychiatric hospital utilize its control and, relatedly, limit its misuse. With regard to the latter, token systems generally place a premium on being open and clear about what is done for each patient. Active attempts by the staff of a token economy to be explicit and public about the procedures they employ help to reduce the probability of their being used naively or maliciously.

This chapter has attempted to identify and to examine the primary characteristic of the token economy approach. Therefore, a discussion of typical intervention procedures, the importance of observing and recording behavior as well as the events affecting it, the necessity for having a well trained staff and an overview of issues central to behavior modification in general has ensued. Token economies are systematic approaches emanating from laboratory developed principles, that can be influential in ameliorating patients' behavior problems. Basic to these systems are the following: (a) listing a variety of relevant behaviors whose performance yields designated numbers of tokens, (b) dispensing tokens, contingent on the occurrences of these desired behaviors, (c) specifying a large number of back-up reinforcers, including commodities, activities, and accommodations, that are exchangeable for specified numbers of tokens, (d) recording all aspects of every token transaction (e.g., what the patient did to receive or forfeit tokens, who were the administrators of tokens, etc.), and keeping data on the total earnings and savings of each patient.

Incorporating mainly principles derived from operant conditioning, token economies are approaches to patient care within a hospital that possess characteristics of a reactive environment; namely, they focus on the patient's behaviors and the context in which they occur, are capable of tailoring treatment variables to the patient's specific needs, provide nonpsychiatric hospital personnel with major responsibility for patient care, are behavioral, and are rehabilitative seeking to ameliorate the patient's behavior problems. Coupled with the determination to broaden its range of influence to the outside environment, the token economy can be an instrument that helps the patient both regain and keep his status as a functioning member of society. The token economy no longer can be denigrated as ineffective or malevolent, but rather must be seen as useful and humane.

It presents an optimistic approach to helping patients behave more capably. It currently is growing in popularity and with much needed research, will be maintained as an attractive treatment modality utilized by an ever growing number of hospital psychiatrists.

Part III

SPECIFIC PROCEDURES IN A REACTIVE ENVIRONMENT

WHEREAS THE PREVIOUS SECTION described the theory and practice of selected unit-wide programs, part III discusses those specific procedures that can be applied and integrated within a psychiatric hospital. The subsequent chapters will examine the admission process, individual psychotherapy, behavior modification, the use of psychotropic agents, activities therapy, group methods, family involvement, and aftercare planning. In discussing these specific procedures we will not present a list of "how-to-do-it" techniques, but rather elucidate the fundamental principles of these various treatment methods. Based on the conviction that many outpatient therapeutic techniques need modification when utilized with hospitalized individuals, part III will discuss specific procedures *only* as they relate to inpatient care. Collectively, these procedures will be examined with a special focus on how they can facilitate observation, evaluation, treatment, and successful aftercare planning.

Chapter 7

THE ADMISSION PROCESS

THE ACT OF BEING ADMITTED to a psychiatric hospital is an important, even tumultuous, event in an individual's lifetime. For some the experience may symbolize the nadir of one's failures, while for others it may represent a welcomed escape from the overwhelming adversities of daily living. Regardless of how the experience of being admitted is perceived, its vital meaning to the patient can hardly be underestimated. In 1970 alone over 598,000 Americans entered psychiatric hospitals (Journal of the American Hospital Association 1971). Despite this, in reviewing the major texts on hospital psychiatry we have been struck by the lack of any in-depth discussion of the admission process. Instead, what one usually encounters is at best a passing reference, and at worst a total avoidance of the subject. This oversight may reflect a general attitude among many hospital psychiatrists who often tend to overlook its tremendous importance to the patient and take the admission process for granted. This is unfortunate, since the patient's initial experience in the hospital may establish a precedent for the events to follow during the course of hospitalization (Greenblatt 1963, Engle 1971, Maxmen 1973b). Therefore, it would seem imperative that any book on hospital practice must include a discussion of the admission process.

FACTORS AFFECTING PSYCHIATRIC HOSPITAL ADMISSION

It is apparent that a multiplicity of factors coalesce in determining how particular individuals come to be admitted to a psychiatric hospital. Although extensive and conclusive research is still needed, certain admission parameters have been identified and are worthy of consideration. For instance, psychiatric inpatients differ from the normal population in that they are older (Department of Health, Education, and Welfare 1972), from cities, and are more likely to be female, non-married, and relatively better educated (Wanklin 1955). Lower socio-economic class patients are disproportionately admitted to state hospitals for both acute treatment and custodial care. On the other hand upper class patients are sent to state institutions only as a "last resort" (Hollingshead 1958).

Numerous authors have postulated that a patient's admission results from a change in his family dynamics (Clausen 1955, Lichtenberg 1960, Pao 1960, Stancer 1965). In a study of 48 Veterans Administration admissions Wood and his collaborators (1960) subdivided patients into a "family group" in which relatives initiated the request for admission, and a "patient group" in which the request came from the patient himself. In the former group it was discovered that the family's demand for a change in the patient's behavior precipitated the hospitalization. In the latter group the patient chose to go to the hospital in order to extricate himself from a disturbing home situation. Another study demonstrated that the more supportive the environment, the less likely the patient is to be hospitalized (Mendel 1969). And finally, with the increasing awareness of family dynamics several authors have even recommended admitting not only the labeled patient, but also the entire family (Bowen 1965, Abroms 1971b).

Mendel and Rapport (1969) have offered statistical evidence suggesting that the staff's administrative procedures and professional experience are more likely to influence the decision to admit than the severity of the patient's presenting behavior. The authors demonstrated that relatively inexperienced psychiatric residents admit more often than experienced ones, and that social workers hospitalize fewer patients than psychiatrists. They also found that admission rates were proportionately higher during evenings and weekends, when this less experienced staff were on duty. It is also known by many psychiatrists that *some* admissions may be determined more by sociopolitical pressure than by psychological need (Weintraub 1964). Although recognizing that social and demographic parameters do influence which patients enter the hospital, others have shown that the patient's actual symptoms are the most critical factors in determining if he is hospitalized (E. Linn 1960, N. Jones 1965).

The expectations of the patient are also important considerations. Various investigators have shown that patients do not enter a hospital with a monolithic set of expectations or attitudes. Instead, they attribute many different meanings to the prospect of being admitted, and anticipate that a wide variety of things will be done to them (L. S. Linn 1968). Those who come to a state hospital with positive expectations more often are male, from broken marriages, from large urban areas, and diagnosed as alcoholic. They are more frequently brought to the hospital by friends or under their own initiative. Conversely, those with negative expectations tend to be female, married, from small rural areas, and non-alcoholic. Furthermore, the patients who are coerced into hospitalization, especially by family members, tend to have an unfavorable predisposition toward being admitted. Patient attitudes regarding hospitalization are not significantly related to their age, educational background, or occupation. Nevertheless, there is a tendency for those who are younger, better educated, and with higher job status to have more negative feelings about being admitted (L. S. Linn 1969).

ADMISSION CRITERIA

Although the main thrust of research points to many factors that are considered in admitting patients, there are comparatively few studies or guidelines as to specific admission criteria. In practice such criteria are usually highly subjective and, therefore, poorly defined. As a result, some individuals are admitted simply because the referring therapist or family wants to get rid of them (C. G. Smith 1972). At other times mental health workers view hospitalization as a last ditch effort when "everything else has failed." When reviewing such cases of "hospitalization by default," it is not unusual to conclude that admitting a patient at an earlier stage of his problem could have prevented a great deal of suffering for both the patient and his family (Group for the Advancement of Psychiatry 1969). At other times half-way houses, drug treatment centers, home visits (Pasamanick 1967), outpatient family-crisis therapy (Langsley 1971), or day hospitalization (Herz 1971) may be useful alternatives to hospitalization (see Greenblatt 1963).

Table VII enumerates a series of reasons which are, we feel, valid indications for admission. Although these criteria may be useful in deciding who should be hospitalized, they do have certain limitations in that they fail to suggest guide lines for determining which patient should be admitted to which facility. We feel that differential admission criteria are necessary for two reasons: (a) different patients have different needs and (b) each hospital can only provide a certain type of rehabilitative program. Contrary to what some mental health professionals may believe, all hospitals cannot provide all kinds of services to all kinds of patients. Therefore, in making the decision to hospitalize someone

TABLE VII

Reasons for Hospitalization

I. Hospitalization for evaluation purposes includes:

 A. extended and careful observation of the patient's behavior

 B. execution of diagnostic procedures such as arteriograms, pneumoencephalograms, and neuropsychiatric testing, that for medical or financial reasons cannot be performed on an outpatient basis.

II. Hospitalization for rehabilitation is indicated when:

 A. varied ambulatory measures have been unsuccessful in halting or reversing the serious maladaptive activities of the patient. This includes instances where suicidal behavior is an immediate threat.

 B. the magnitude of a patient's regressive, depressive, anti social, or aggressive behavior is no longer tolerable to those in the environment.

 C. the execution of special procedures, such as ECT, cannot be performed on an outpatient basis.

 D. alcohol or drugs upon which the patient has become dependent cannot be safely withdrawn on an outpatient basis.

 E. the administration of medication would be too dangerous to be carried out as an outpatient.

 F. the behavioral components of an incapacitating medical illness cannot be handled optimally on a medical or surgical service.

III. Hospitalization as a prophylactic measure may be useful in order to:

 A. motivate a patient and/or his family to accept and to support the therapeutic efforts of the outpatient therapist.

 B. remove the patient from a psychonoxious environment, so that an exploration and resolution of his critical relationships can proceed before a crisis emerges.

 C. readminister drugs to an uncooperative patient for whom the likelihood of serious maladaptive behavior would be highly probable unless medication is restarted.

we feel that ideally it would be helpful to have precise criteria for admitting a particular patient to a specific hospital.

Although many diverse parameters could be utilized in constructing a set of differential admission criteria, we believe the following may provide some practical guidelines for hospital personnel.

1. *Indications for Short-term Hospitalization* (less than 3 weeks).

(a) *All types of evaluation* can be performed in a short-term facility. Thus, if a patient is referred to a hospital for evaluation *only*, we feel it should be carried out in a short-term setting. (b) *Treatment* should occur in a short-term facility if the patient has suffered an acute deterioration of his behavior. We define "acute" somewhat arbitrarily, as meaning within the last six months. By this we do not wish to imply that the patient was without difficulties prior to a half a year ago, but rather that his *presenting* problem began within a six-month period. Since problems of recent onset more readily respond to brief inpatient treatment (e.g. Vaillant 1964), we feel that short-term hospitalization is preferable for such individuals.

2. *Indications for Intermediate-term Hospitalization* (three weeks to six months).

(a) Patients who fail to respond to treatment in a short-term hospital should be referred to an intermediate-term facility, assuming that alternatives to hospitalization such as half-way houses are neither available nor desirable. We do not believe that patients with an acute problem should be directly transferred from a short-term to a long-term unit, since hospitalization in our estimation should be as brief as possible. (b) Patients with a "chronic" (more than six months) deterioration of behavior should be initially referred to an intermediate-term hospital. Because these patients are unlikely to respond within a three-week period, hospitalization in a short-term facility would be ill-advised, since in all probability these patients would eventually need to be transferred to an intermediate-term facility anyway. The only exception to this is when prior to admission it is understood that the patient is primarily being hospitalized for a trial of electro-convulsive treatment. In these cases a short-term hospital would be preferable.

3. *Indications for a Long-term Hospitalization* (greater than six months).

Patients who fail to respond to intermediate-term hospitalization should go to a long-term unit, unless alternative non-hospital facilities such as drug treatment centers are available and desirable. We do not feel, as some do (Hilles 1970, Kernberg 1973), that any patient should have an initial hospitalization in a long-term treatment center.

GOALS OF ADMISSION PROCEDURES

Even though it is generally acknowledged that a patient's first impression of a hospital may have a significant impact on the outcome of his treatment, the procedures used for admitting him have oftentimes been taken for granted. In order to avoid this it is useful for hospital staff to develop admission procedures with clearly defined goals.

When screening an applicant for hospitalization, we have also found that it is advisable to consult with the significant people in the patient's social environment. The initial task of such a meeting is to gather only as much history as will be necessary to determine if the patient should be admitted. The criteria found in Table VII may be of assistance in reaching this decision.

Once having decided to admit the patient, in all but the most emergent situations, the remainder of this meeting can be devoted to accomplishing the following objectives:

1. *Providing an orientation.* It is helpful to orient the patient and, if available, his family to the hospital's treatment philosophy and program. This may help in allaying anxieties over the prospect of hospitalization.

2. *Defining and adjusting expectations.* In order to minimize

misunderstanding, the patient and his relatives ought to clarify what they expect from hospitalization. In turn the staff can indicate if they feel they are able to reasonably meet these expectations. If not, this may be noted, and a more feasible contract may be arranged.

3. *Collecting a data base.* It may be valuable to provide the patient and his family with a set of self-administered comprehensive questionnaires. These forms, which contain questions about a patient's personal, family, and psychiatric history, may be returned to the staff on the day of admission.

4. *Obtaining release of information form.* This is helpful in order to collect data from other treatment facilities with which the patient has had prior contract. Ideally, this information should be sent for early enough so that it becomes available to the hospital staff on the day of admission.

Once the patient is admitted to the hospital, the staff is faced with two important tasks. The first is to acquire a complete *history* from the patient and those significant individuals comprising his social network. The major purpose of the admission history is to determine which, if any, further psychological, social, or medical evaluations need to be performed in order to institute an effective treatment plan. It is also important to determine those specific behaviors that interfere with the patient's current functioning, his diagnosis, the factors within his previous environment that may have contributed to his present difficulties, and who, if anyone, in the patient's social network should be involved in the treatment program.

The second important task of the hospital staff is to facilitate the newly admitted patient's *adaptation* to the unit. Staff, as well as patients, can be of assistance in acquainting the new arrival with the unit's personnel and programs. Specific techniques for accomplishing this, as well as other aspects of the total admission process, can be found elsewhere (Grant 1971, Maxmen 1973b).

In conclusion the literature on the process of admitting a patient to a psychiatric unit suggests that a mixture of factors contribute to deciding which patients are admitted to which hospitals. We have suggested criteria for admitting patients to particular facilities. Finally, the goals of the admitting process have been examined. Once having entered the hospital the patient encounters a highly complex system to which we now turn our attention.

Chapter 8

THE HOSPITAL AS A SYSTEM

WHEN THE PATIENT is admitted to a psychiatric hospital, he enters a complex task system[1]. How this structured system interacts with the patient may to a large extent determine if hospitalization becomes a therapeutic experience for him. Conversely, the behavior of patients may affect the structure and staff of a unit. Thus, the patients, staff, and structure of a psychiatric hospital exist in a dynamic equilibrium, each influencing the others.

There are, of course, variables emanating from beyond the walls of a hospital which affect the patients, staff, and structure of a psychiatric unit. These parameters include political, economic, and cultural considerations. For example, the method of financing health care greatly influences the quality of psychiatric treatment and the eligibility of patients to avail themselves of it.

Although such extra-mural factors significantly affect the prac-

---

[1] A system can be defined as "a complex of interacting elements" (Bertalanffy 1968, p. 55). A task system can be defined as "a system of activities plus the human and physical resources required to perform the activities" (Miller 1967, p. 6). General systems theorists believe that it is impossible to fully understand an organizational system by exclusively examining its parts.

tice of hospital psychiatry we shall confine our discussion to those variables within the unit that influence the hospital system. More specifically, we will examine the treatment objectives of the hospital, the general principles of the particular treatment methods utilized in order to accomplish these goals, and several circumstances that may interfere with or even disrupt the system from attaining these objectives.

GOALS OF A HOSPITAL SYSTEM

At the most general level the objectives of a hospital system are to minimize problematic behaviors and to impart useful skills. Abroms (1968, 1969b) has listed five general types of unadaptive behaviors that need to be minimized in order to enable patients to successfully leave the hospital.

1. *Destructiveness*. This includes suicidal, homicidal, assaultive, self-mutilative, and other forms of physically destructive behavior.

2. *Disorganization*. This refers to a large range of behaviors usually associated with psychotic disorders, such as hallucinations, delusions, disorientation, incoherent speech, and bizarre activity.

3. *Deviancy or Rule Breaking Behavior*. This refers to what has been loosely termed "acting-up" behavior, such as drug abuse, promiscuity, violence, and stealing.

4. *Dysphoria*. This includes symptoms of depression, mania, social withdrawal, agitation, and phobias.

5. *Dependency*. This refers to a general class of behaviors, all of which involve the patient's transferring responsibility for his conduct and care onto others.

Abroms feels that the order of these five D's of maladaptive behaviors suggests not only their relative severity, but also provides a list of priorities for determining treatment interventions. Thus, a hospital staff must first contend with the destructive behavior of the patient before attempting to alleviate his dysphoric activity. Similarly, the patient's deviant behavior should be minimized before dealing with his dependency strivings.

Although it is easy for the hospital staff to focus on decreasing problematic behaviors, the expansion of the patient's useful activities must not be forgotten. Depending on the requirements of the particular patient, any or all of the following areas may need to be taught.

1. *Interpersonal skills.* These include a wide range of abilities, such as being able to converse with others, to be assertive, and to recognize social nuances. Interpersonal skills are useful for the adequate performance of the next three categories of behavior.

2. *Occupational Skills.* These include marketable activities, such as running a machine, cleaning a house, driving a bus, keeping to a schedule, and organizing one's work habits.

3. *Recreational Skills.* These refer to acquiring the ability to enjoy leisure time with or without the presence of others. Being able to select recreational activities, feeling comfortable participating in them, allotting time for such activities, etc., are all important areas to be taught in such a program.

4. *Health Maintenance Skills.* This general class of behaviors includes the hospitalized patient's ability to recognize situations that may lead to future distress, to establish a hierarchy of treatment issues, to understand the possible biological factors that influence his problems, and to be sensitive to potential danger signals of an impending behavioral decompensation.

Before attempting to minimize problematic behaviors and to strengthen adaptive skills the staff and the patient should agree, whenever possible, on the behaviors that should be altered. In other words under ideal circumstances there should be a mutual understanding between the staff and the patient as to the goals of hospitalization. This agreement, however, does not preclude the possibility that treatment objectives may be revised as hospitalization proceeds. In reaching such a contract it may be necessary for the staff to help the patient identify his problematic behaviors (Davies 1970, Detre 1971b). Novice therapists may feel reluctant to do so, believing that they will embarrass the patient, and thereby aggravate his condition. At other times a therapist may avoid giving a patient honest feedback about his behavior in order to shield himself from the anger of the patient. In both of these circumstances the staff may fail to discuss the patient's maladaptive activities with him, preferring either to present the patient with an elaborate formulation of his problems, limit conversation to issues of medication, or simply ignore the patient altogether. By avoiding an open discussion of the patient's most obvious difficulties, however, the therapist inadvertently conveys the message that the patient is "too sick" to tolerate direct communication. In turn the patient's symptoms may be aggravated because he correctly perceives that he being treated with "kid gloves." We feel that it is preferable to help the patient recognize his problematic behaviors so that he learns to alter them and to acquire health maintenance skills. The major point is, however, that the establishment of a treatment contract helps the staff determine how the patient and the hospital system should interact.

While establishing a contract between the patient and the staff, hospital personnel should be alert to the possibility that the goals of the patient may *reasonably* differ from those of the hospital system. For example, a patient was admitted to the hospital and vigorously treated for her chronic visual hallucinations. As the hallucinations subsided, the patient became increasingly hostile towards the staff. After considerable turmoil, it was discovered that the patient did not wish to relinquish her hallucinations because they "had always kept her company." Further discussion revealed that although the staff wanted to minimize her perceptual disorder, the patient only desired to improve her marriage. Thus, hospitalization and the turmoil that had transpired during a large portion of it may have been avoided, if the staff had not just *assumed* that it knew what the patient had desired (see Lazare 1972).

THE USE OF SPECIFIC TREATMENT MODALITIES

Whatever the particular treatment goals may happen to be, many patients can attain these objectives solely by participating in unit-wide programs, such as a therapeutic community or a token economy. For other patients, however, additional specific treatment modalities (e.g. individual, group, or family therapies) may need to be added to the patient's unit-wide program in order to enhance and to facilitate his rehabilitation. We feel that these *supplemental* treatment procedures should be *specifically* prescribed according to the individual needs of the patient. When prescribing medication, this principle is usually adhered to; depressed patients are generally given anti-depressants, schizophrenic patients are usually given phenothiazines, and other patients are given no medication at all. Nevertheless, hospital staff tend to be less selective when prescribing other treatment techniques; they tend to offer a therapeutic modality merely because that modality exists or because it "can't hurt" anyone. Therefore, even though nobody would suggest that every patient should take phenothiazines, oftentimes individual or group therapy are automatically prescribed for everybody.

In conceptualizing the role of specific treatment modalities in a hospital system two unsatisfactory frameworks seem to prevail. In some facilities one particular treatment technique, such as individual or group psychotherapy, occupies center stage, the rest of the program being arranged to enhance the favored treatment procedure. In other hospitals numerous distinct therapies are provided, each being afforded relatively equal significance, but none of them appearing to have any relationship to one another; as a result a meaningless eclecticism prevails that is devoid of any overall conceptual framework. Instead, as indicated in chapter 3, we would propose a third alternative; namely, that every specific treatment procedure within a psychiatric hospital should exist in a dynamic equilibrium with one another as well as with the unit's overall program.

Because the hospital must be viewed as a system, what transpires during the application of any one specific treatment procedure affects to some extent what will occur during every other one. Thus, the utilization of a particular treatment modality cannot be viewed as existing in isolation. For example, somebody who conducts individual psychotherapy should know what happens during his patient's group therapy as well as during other experiences the patient encounters within the hospital. In a group therapy meeting a patient hinted he would run away from the unit. Later in an individual psychotherapy session the doctor, unaware of the patient's comments in the earlier group meeting, proceeded to discuss issues that arose in his previous session with the patient. The latter, hoping the doctor would persuade him to stay, became increasingly agitated as the therapist failed to discuss his threat of running away. Believing that the psychiatrist did not care about him, the patient fled from the hospital. This unfortunate situation may have been averted, if the doctor had known what the patient had said during group therapy. Thus, in order for the staff to utilize specific treatment modalities effectively, the unit needs to have a mechanism by which information from varied hospital programs or experiences can be integrated. Failure to do so can prevent the hospital system from attaining its objectives.

DISRUPTIONS OF THE SYSTEM

There are, of course, many circumstances that may prevent or disrupt the hospital system from accomplishing its goals. Poorly trained staff, cumbersome administrative procedures, a change of therapists, the admission of a V.I.P. (Weintraub 1964), deleterious interference by those not involved in the hospital program, etc., all can serve to attenuate the effectiveness of inpatient treatment. It is not the purpose of this book to discuss every set of behaviors or situations that can potentially disrupt the psychiatric hospital. Nevertheless, two distinct and frequently occurring disruptions are worthy of comment, namely, acting-up[1] and the "Special Patient" syndrome.

---

[1] We feel the term acting-up is more descriptive than the frequently used term "acting-out"; the latter implies an etiological explanation based on the notion of transference.

Acting-up

By the term acting-up we include a wide range of behaviors from minor rule breaking to major transgressions of socially accepted standards of conduct—all of which either offend or disrupt other individuals in the patient's social sphere. Under the rubric of acting-up behaviors are activities such as taking illegal drugs, committing violence, running away, or encouraging other patients to transgress.

Prevention of these types of behaviors requires prompt diagnosis and treatment. For the most part patients who act-up in the hospital have done so prior to being admitted. Initial assessment data should alert the staff to these potential difficulties. Also, it is necessary to forecast situations that tend to provoke anti-social behavior. A change of therapists, an impending discharge, a potentially explosive family visit—the consequences of all of these events should be anticipated so the staff can make appropriate interventions. Conversely, overlooking anti-social behavior may encourage even further acting-up. Thus, hospital personnel can usually prevent these behaviors by anticipating them rather than by merely responding to them.

In treating such problems the ultimate goal is to help the patient develop self-control. Nevertheless, until internal controls are developed, hospital personnel may need to take charge; a staff that fails to do so abdicates its therapeutic responsibility. McDonald (1965) has offered six important guidelines that may assist staff in minimizing acting-up behavior.

1. *Set as few limits as possible.* Patients resent too many restrictions and nurses find them a nuisance to remember and especially to enforce. The more limits that are set, the more likely some of them will be unjust.

2. *Clearly define limits.* Specificity, clarity, and simplicity are necessary in setting limits if the staff is to avoid ambiguous interpretations of the restrictions. Acting-up patients seem to relish the opportunity to exploit different interpretations of the rules. Furthermore, ambiguity on the part of hospital personnel can gen-

erate a sense of frustration and injustice in the patient, leading to even further acting-up (see Marohn 1973).

3. *Limits explained to the patient should be understood by the staff.* It is important that the restrictions told to the patient are identical to those on the order sheet.

4. *Limits should be enforceable.* For example, it is impractical to allow a patient to have dinner outside of the hospital, but insist that he cannot have an alcoholic beverage.

5. *Enforce limits promptly.* At least in the initial stage of hospitalization failure to respond immediately to the patient's deviant behavior encourages further acting-up. Whether the response consists of merely serving a warning or reducing privileges, it should follow the event promptly. If a time lag ensues, the patient may have difficulty recognizing that the punishment is in response to his misbehavior. Also, by not immediately setting limits the patient may believe that the staff is unconcerned about his maladaptive behavior.

6. *Give sound reasons for limits.* Sometimes the wrong reasons are given for the right restrictions. A patient with a history of persistently surreptitious alcohol abuse was confined to the unit. Rather than saying that the reason for setting this limit was that it was routine hospital policy, it would have been preferable for the therapist to tell the patient that, at least temporarily, the staff felt he was unreliable. Furthermore, by offering an honest and sensible reason for restrictions a therapist may stimulate valuable discussion regarding the patient's major behavior problems. And finally, after giving the patient a sound reason for the restrictions, it is advisable for staff members to avoid becoming embroiled in lengthy and unproductive debates with the patient about the legitimacy of the limit setting. Frequently, the longer these arguments ensue, the more the acting-up patients can play upon the ambivalent feelings of the therapist and manipulate the staff.

In setting limits several other principles should be considered. After setting limits, the staff must be prepared to endure the patient's transitory hostility. It should be remembered that despite a patient's frequent protestations about being restricted, limits may be necessary, at least temporarily, until the patient behaves more appropriately. On the other hand reasonable requests by an acting-up patient should not be *automatically* refused merely because the therapist feels he is being manipulated. If a request is denied, it should be done so for legitimate reasons. And finally, limit setting oftentimes engenders hostility not only in the patient who acts-up, but in other patients as well. Because the psychiatric unit is a system in which the actions of one influence the responses of all, limit setting cannot be carried out optimally without the involvement of the entire hospital community. By portraying themselves as innocent victims or by spreading vindictive rumors, those who act-up may provoke the staff to fight among themselves or with the other patients. If limits are to be set, ideally the entire staff and patient community should be consulted beforehand in order to ascertain information and to share the reasons for the restrictions (see chapter 5). Failure to do so can lead to acting-up by other patients as well as by other staff.

One type of acting-up patient who deserves special attention is the one who threatens or commits acts of violence. Although seriously violent behavior is a rare event among hospitalized individuals (Kalogerakis 1971) the spectre of violence arouses intense anxiety in both patients and staff. As a result, hospital personnel tend to overreact to patients who demonstrate a propensity towards assaultive behavior. Lion and Pasternak (1973) have described situations in which hospital staff (a) exaggerate the dangerousness of potentially violent patients, (b) avoid conversing with them about their threatening behavior, (c) deny their propensity to commit dangerous acts, or (d) treat them in an excessively punitive fashion.

Even though hospital personnel may overreact to the potentially assaultive patient, threatening behavior should not be treated lightly. Several authors have stressed the importance of routinely asking all newly admitted patients about a previous history of violent acts, the presence of paranoid delusions, the ownership of weapons, the possession of lethal skills, etc. (MacDonald 1966, Kalogerakis 1971, Lion 1973). Kalogerakis (1971) found that the presence of other disturbed patients, boredom, overcrowding, staff abuse, and a feeling of being rendered helpless by an overpowering staff may all trigger violent acts in those hospitalized patients who have a propensity toward such behavior. It must be remembered that in most circumstances not only is the staff frightened of violent behavior, but so is the patient himself. Appropriate use of medication, verbal interaction, and limit setting are necessary in order to help the assaultive patient control his own destructive impulses, as well as to protect others who come into contact with him. And finally, other patients in the hospital need to be informed about the presence of the violent patient; more importantly, the staff needs to assist the patient community in learning to help rather than to aggravate the potentially dangerous individual (see chaper 5).

The "Special Patient" Syndrome

In a classic paper on hospital psychiatry T. F. Main (1957) described a clinical phenomenon known as the "Special Patient" syndrome. This paper deserves our attention because it illustrates that information from individual patient contacts should be shared with the entire staff, and that communication among hospital personnel must remain open and forthright. But most importantly, the "Special Patient" syndrome demonstrates how latent intra-staff conflict can be exploited by certain patients, so that ultimately the hospital personnel are in conflict while the patient's behavior degenerates even further.

The Special Patient does not possess any particular demographic or diagnostic characteristics. Nevertheless, staff members can detect his presence, if they are sensitive to certain behaviors of the Patient, unusual responses in themselves, as well as in other hospital personnel. In its most blatant form the "Special Patient" syndrome usually develops as follows. Before admission the referring therapist demonstrates an intense concern for the Patient and may even express the desire that routine admission procedures be circumvented because of the Patient's unusual degree of stress, helplessness, and vulnerability. Oftentimes the history reveals that the Patient has failed to improve despite numerous hospitalizations; the referring therapist feels that intensive therapy is definitely indicated, implying that he knows what is best for the Patient. Self-destructive acts may be viewed by the referrer not as a danger signal, but rather as an indication that others had mishandled his case by being too insensitive, unimaginative, or crude. At the same time relatives seem to feel that other relatives have been unresponsive to the Patient's "real" needs, and frequently become antagonistic towards one another.

After the Patient is admitted, some staff feel their special sensitivity, special devotion, and special concern will compensate for the Patient's previous neglect. "Mere" routines are not going to interfere with their compelling desire to rectify the Patient's former therapeutic deprivation. Special relationships begin to develop between particular staff members and the Patient. These close alliances evolve out of a sense that the Patient's needs are not being met by other hospital personnel, and are confirmed when the Patient confides with a particular staff member some deep dark secret which allegedly he has not told anybody else. The staff member who has been "honored" by receiving this "confidential" comunication begins to develop an exclusive relationship with the Patient based upon the Patient's "sentimental appeal" and the staff member's "arousal of omnipotence." Spurred on by rescue fantasies, certain staff members begin to feel that they alone possess a special sensitivity to the Patient and are the only ones who can possibly administer to his needs. Despite this supposed understanding, the Patient continues to regress; no amount of attention ever seems to satisfy him.

Eventually, many other staff members develop special relationships to the Patient. Insisting upon even more permissiveness, they, even at great personal expense, cater to his every whim. As the Patient's maladaptive activities increase, this is viewed as evidence that the Patient needs more intensive devotion, rather than signalling that the special approach is reinforcing problematic behavior.

Ultimately, this situation leads to a schism among the staff. The "in-group" who are "chosen" by the Patient demand more therapy, more drugs, more attention, more consultations, and more protection from the alleged abuses of other hospital personnel. Even among the in-group there is competition to see who can be the most favored by the Patient. On the other hand the "out-group" are those who do not have a special relationship with the Patient. Although somewhat envious they resent the therapeutic gymnastics of the in-group and increasingly express their displeasure with such activities. They believe the over-indulgence of the in-group allows the Patient to "get away with murder" and, as a result, the out-group either overcompensates by being unusually strict with or totally withdraws from the Patient. This mounting staff conflict may lead to disastrous results, i.e., the Special Patient oftentimes becomes a special failure; he may be transferred to another hospital or eventually commit suicide.

As Main points out, the Special Patient transforms covert staff conflict into overt intra-staff antagonism. It is only by carefully diagnosing the "Special Patient" syndrome and by openly acknowledging one's involvement in the phenomenon that a staff can provide a constructive treatment program for the Patient. When staff finds itself unwilling to share with other hospital personnel secrets divulged to them by patients, the "Special Patient" syndromes in its less overt manifestations may be developing.

The phenomenon of the "Special Patient" syndrome underscores the necessity to view the hospital as a system. The interaction between a single staff member and the Patient may yield consequences that extend far beyond that particular relationship; to some extent, every staff member, every patient, and every program may be affected. In turn these changes lead to even further modifications of the hospital system. Ultimately, these changes may distract or even prevent the psychiatric hospital from attaining its objectives. In order to avoid these deleterious consequences, as well as to enhance everyone's rehabilitative efforts, the staff must regulate the hospital system by the judicious use of unit-wide programs and specific treatment modalities. Although each of the following chapters will separately examine specific treatment procedures these separations are in reality somewhat arbitrary divisions, because the hospital is a system; what transpires in each treatment session affects what occurs in every other one. This principle is of vital significance to all those who seek to provide psychiatric treatment to hospitalized individuals.

Chapter 9

INDIVIDUAL PROCEDURES: PSYCHOTHERAPY AND BEHAVIOR MODIFICATION

AMONG THE MOST IMPORTANT treatment techniques utilized in a psychiatric hospital are what we shall call "individual procedures." By this term we mean those therapies that are *specifically convened* and brought to bear on particular problems of certain individual patients. These approaches are to be distinguished somewhat arbitrarily from other treatment modalities, such as activities, group, and family therapies. As with every other type of specific treatment technique, individual procedures are to be prescribed specifically for a particular patient in order to *supplement* the hospital's unit-wide program.

There are numerous types of individual procedures that may need to be included in the patient's treatment program. Certainly, many psychiatric inpatients suffer from medical problems that interfere with their physical health and behavioral functioning. The increasing establishment of psychiatric units within general hospitals, as well as our expanding understanding of the biological influences on mental illness, has served to underscore the physician's vital role in the treatment of certain patients. Thus, one type of individual procedure involves attending to the particular medical needs of hospitalized patients.

Another significant individual procedure is the selective use of psychopharmacologic agents. Because of the important role of medication in the treatment of hospitalized individuals, this subject will be discussed in the following chapter.

In this section we will examine two other common types of individual procedures; namely, dyadic psychotherapy and individually-directed behavior modification programs. In discussing these methods we will primarily outline the general principles of their utilization within a hospital, rather than provide a compendium of specific treatment techniques.

PSYCHOTHERAPY

In this chapter psychotherapy will be defined as a psychological process between two people in which the therapist by virtue of his position, training, and knowledge attempts to systematically apply, mainly through verbal interchange, certain psychological principles and techniques in order to modify a patient's behavior. There are, of course, numerous schools of psychotherapy, such as Freudian, Jungian, Adlerian, Sullivanian, Rogerian, Kaiserian, etc. Regardless of one's particular theoretical persuasion we maintain that the use of these therapies with psychiatric outpatients needs to be altered when applied to hospitalized individuals.

Because of psychotherapy's preeminent status in American psychiatry, the professional literature is focused almost exclusively on devising methods to alter the hospital's milieu in order to facilitate the practice of psychotherapy (e.g. Rinsley 1968, Gralnick 1969a, Garber 1972). To a large extent this approach is backwards. In chapter 3 we stated that ideally the hour of psychotherapy between the doctor and the patient should be as important as any other hour on the unit. Therefore, *it would seem preferable to modify our psychotherapeutic techniques in order to potentiate the overall effectiveness of the total hospital program, rather than to modify the total program in order to potentiate the use of psy-*

chotherapy. In many facilities psychotherapy is viewed as the "real" therapy, while everything else appears to be merely "supportive" or "what you do until the doctor comes." When *the* doctor does arrive, he sequesters himself with the patient in order to conduct *the* psychotherapy, without ever sharing with other staff members the content of the session. This method of operation is not only demeaning to other hospital personnel, but prevents the staff from working in a unified and consistent manner.

Instead, we would suggest that the *content of individual psychotherapy within a hospital setting should consist primarily of information derived from the in-hospital behavior of the patient.* Once he has been admitted, it is the continuation of the patient's maladaptive behaviors within the hospital that prevents him from being discharged. Therefore, because hospitalization is an abnormal human activity, treatment must be directed toward rectifying this abnormal situation by mainly focusing upon the problematic behaviors that are currently responsible for the patient's continued presence within a psychiatric unit.

Because the hospital provides a total living situation in which the patient's activities can be observed throughout the day, the psychotherapist is afforded the unique opportunity to acquire information usually not available to his outpatient colleagues. Failure to utilize this source of data minimizes the potential advantages of psychotherapy with hospitalized individuals. Furthermore, the therapist can determine if his psychotherapeutic intervention is having the desired effect by observing whether the patient's behavior is improving on the unit. In this way the milieu can provide feedback to the therapist. If the patient's maladaptive behaviors continue, the therapist should then consider altering his treatment approach. All too often therapists assume that a patient's improvement in individual psychotherapy generalizes to the unit. Oftentimes this is not the case. A delinquent adolescent may appear to be making positive strides in psychotherapy, but continues to wreak havoc everywhere else. If the psychotherapist discounts or ignores this anti-social activity as merely the result of a "difficult stage in therapy," he may be undermining not only the patient's progress, but also the efforts of the entire staff. By making the in-hospital behavior of the patient the primary data for individual psychotherapy the doctor helps to reduce the possibility of a schism among the staff. The therapist may no longer view the hospital personnel as meddling in his psychotherapy; conversely, the staff may no longer view the psychotherapist as being unconcerned with their treatment efforts.

By focusing on in-hospital behavior the therapist helps the patient to understand the transactional impact of his activity on others and attempts to suggest alternative methods of adapting. One way to attain these objectives is for the psychotherapist to show the patient that some of his behavior within the hospital closely resembles the activity that has been or will be deemed unacceptable by others in the community. For example, a suicidal patient was admitted to the hospital after her husband threatened divorce. Although her spouse accused her of philandering, the patient vehemently proclaimed her unswerving devotion to her husband. In the course of hospitalization it was frequently noted that the patient flirted with many of the male staff members. During an individual psychotherapy session the psychiatrist pointed out her coquettish behavior on the unit, suggested that it seemed to resemble her activity with men outside the hospital, and that it possibly contributed to her husband's wish to terminate the marriage. In this example the psychiatrist helped the patient become more aware of her in-hospital behavior and suggested to her that it may have contributed to her marital difficulties prior to admission.

In conducting psychotherapy with hospitalized individuals historical data is of value *only* to the extent that it clarifies the patient's current activity and leads to more useful behaviors. Similarly, psychodynamic exploration in and of itself is meaningless, unless it generates adaptive strivings within the total hospital milieu.

If the patient fails to be involved in the daily activities of the unit, the therapist will be unable to fully utilize the data from the patient's in-hospital behavior as a source of information for the psychotherapeutic hour. Thus, it is incumbent on the psychotherapist to encourage the patient to participate actively in all aspects of the hospital's treatment program that are deemed important to the patient's rehabilitation (Davies 1970). For example, if a socially isolated patient has failed to come to group therapy, the individual therapist may wish to help the patient identify those specific aspects of the group situation that the patient seems to be avoiding. This avoidance of group may be explored with the aim of showing how it relates to the patient's more general problem with social isolation. On the other hand, if the therapist limits discussion to events of the distant past or the distant future, psychotherapy becomes a sterile enterprise. It fails to contend with the patient's immediate problems in the hospital, thereby divorcing psychotherapy from other aspects of the unit's program. In whatever way it will be helpful the therapist must encourage the patient's participation in those hospital programs which are believed to be beneficial to the patient. By witnessing his therapist's active participation in the unit the patient, perhaps by means of identification, may be encouraged to become involved in the program himself. Consequently, the therapist also needs to be an integral part of the unit's activity, if he is to avail himself of the in-hospital data.

By focusing primarily on the activity the patient demonstrates in the unit the therapist is still left with the task of transferring adaptive behaviors in the hospital to settings outside of it. Our experience coincides with that of Davies and Coughlin (1970), who maintain that patients who are unable to generalize positive behaviors from the psychotherapeutic session to the rest of the unit are rarely able to demonstrate useful activities in the community. In other words patients have a better chance of coping successfully with life outside the hospital, if they are able to initially demonstrate constructive behavior inside of it. Once the latter is accomplished, psychotherapy must then turn its attention to the realities patients will face after discharge. This may include a discussion of those adaptive skills that the patient lacks which will be necessary for him to attain before leaving the hospital. Generally speaking, at the outset of hospitalization, the psychotherapist may need to focus on minimizing problematic behaviors. During the latter stages therapy may need to focus on transmitting adaptive skills. The point is that as hospitalization proceeds, the therapeutic emphasis may need modification.

BEHAVIOR MODIFICATION PROGRAMS

The principles of behavior modification that are applicable to individuals in a psychiatric hospital can fill a textbook; to attempt here in a few pages to illustrate all these procedures would be impossible. Instead, we will offer a few examples of how behavior modification can be implemented for an individual patient. Although behavioral practices, such as systematic desensitization, behavioral rehearsal, and assertive training (Wolpe 1969), are capable of being applied in a psychiatric hospital, we shall limit our discussion to methods derived from operant conditioning. Although these latter techniques have been used effectively in short-term facilities (R. C. Smith 1972), more frequently they have been applied in the treatment of intermediate and long-term patients. The following report illustrates such an example.

Cockrill and Bernal (1968) reported a case in which a withdrawn patient was helped via a behavior modification approach to begin conversations in a dyadic interaction. The study was technically sophisticated and was presented in the literature as an experimental and somewhat novel treatment; it represents a beginning step in the development of a more extensive behavioral intervention. Two of its most significant aspects were that another patient acted as therapist in carrying the treatment out, and that a psychiatric nurse designed and orchestrated it. The study proceeded through four stages: baseline, intervention, return to baseline, and return to intervention. Twelve 15-minute sessions, three times per week for one month, were required to execute the program. Both the withdrawn patient (target patient) and the patient-therapist were roommates and had established, previous to the program, some degree of rapport. The target behavior was the patient initiating a verbal interchange. The target patient and the patient-therapist were to generate a conversation over a picture that was given to them. Both were instructed to compose a story about the picture or to discuss anything it suggested. Baseline recordings consisted of what each patient did in response to the other. From the baseline data, definitions of the target behavior and potential positive reinforcers for the target patient were identified. An *initiation* was defined as a "direct question, a request for information, or a statement introducing a new topic." Positive reinforcers for the target patient consisted of behavior of the patient-therapist, namely, "verbal agreement or approval," "smiling or laughing," and "up and down head nods." All this information was garnered from videotapes, but it could have been gathered by direct observation. After five sessions of baseline data collection, the intervention phase began. The patient-therapist was instructed to provide positive reinforcement when the target patient initiated discourse. In order to facilitate the implementation of this contingency the patient-therapist was instructed to reduce her normally frequent initiations to approximately one-fourth of her baseline level. By the end of the three-session intervention stage the patient's initiation behavior increased dramatically. In order to evaluate if the social reinforcement was responsible for the patient's adaptive behavior, the reinforcers were discontinued for two sessions. The resultant drop in the target behavior helped in proving that the total positive reinforcement method was responsible for the improvement. A return to intervention for two more sessions recaptured the high frequency of initiation made by the target patient. No follow-up data were reported.

This study demonstrated that behavior modification was effective in the sense that the target behavior was significantly changed. What happens, however, to the patient after the program ends? This study does not report that behavior modification is meaningful in the sense that the behavior change endures or that desirable behavior occurs in new situations with other patients or staff, or that new socially relevant activities begin to take place. (Baer 1968, LeBow 1973). The issue here is the same one previously brought up for token economies; namely, the importance of fostering durable and generalized behavior changes. As indicated in chapter 6, accomplishing these goals may involve the structuring and restructuring of environments that nurture and support these alterations of behavior. In this study an initial environment, constituted by the target patient and the patient-therapist, was created to begin modification. Another environment to which the positive effects of the previous environment could have been extended is the hospital unit, wherein the target patient, staff, and patient peers interact. In time rehabilitation may continue in other settings such as the patient's home, work, and school situations. As the target patient begins to demonstrate improvement, the artificiality of the technique gradually will be abandoned while more "spontaneous" interactions develop. *The main point is that long-term and extensive behavioral changes are possible, if they are supported by the environment in which the patient behaves.*

It is imperative in all behavior modification programs for individual patients that the activity of the patient serve as one's guide. If the patient fails to improve after a reasonable period of time, then the program needs to be changed. In other words it is incumbent upon the staff to alter the program, rather than to merely accuse the patient of being "unmotivated" or to simply assume the patient is hopelessly incapacitated. Thus, *only* the adaptive responses of the patient determine if a treatment program is successful.

Behavior modification programs for individual patients may be designed by nurses, aides, psychiatrists, psychologists, social workers, etc. But, in contrast to psychotherapy, the persons carrying it out should be the ones who have the most continuous daily contact with the patient. Once established, these programs need not be extremely time-consuming, but they often do require vigilance on the part of the administrator.

A program for a patient can be implemented on or off the unit, depending on the behaviors being modified, the phase of the program being implemented, and the vicissitudes of the situation. Individual behavior modification plans can be applied in an ongoing token economy ward (Schaefer 1969), a therapeutic community (Abroms, 1971a, Grant 1971), or on units run by a different principle (R. C. Smith 1972). Regardless of where the program is being carried out, it is vital that the situation in which it takes place, and the individuals responsible for administering each aspect of it, are specified. To maximize its success, one must gather reliable and extensive observational data throughout the various phases of the program. Before detailed and quantified observations are collected, however, identification and definition of the behavioral difficulties and the situations influencing them must take place. In addition it is valuable to specify potentially positive reinforcers for the patient. As Ludwig (1971) points out, often these reinforcers are not readily apparent and differ from events commonly assumed to be rewards. For instance, tender loving care may fortify, in some patients, *undesirable* ways of acting; also the opportunity to be discharged from the hospital may exacerbate behavior problems. To find out what are a patient's positive reinforcers, ask him, and more importantly, observe him. As mentioned in chapter 6, no substitute exists for empirically verifying what specific events can function as positive reinforcers.

Baseline data, as indicated, provide the staff member with knowledge of the frequency of the behavior problem. When this pre-treatment information shows that a behavioral difficulty is *not* markedly fluctuating from day to day, and is not evidencing any trends towards diminishing "by itself," then intervention procedures may be applied. Ideally, therefore, baseline records should indicate that the target behavior is *stable*. If it is occurring frequently one day and not the next, however, check to see what factors are present during the observation sessions or immediately preceding them that may account for this fluctuation. To begin intervention before one has given the behavior a chance to stabilize or before one has attempted to delineate the possible causes of the fluctuation is unwise. For example, suppose one desires to use a positive reinforcement procedure for a patient who talks incoherently. The baseline data indicate that this incoherence occurs in strength one day but not the next. It would be naive to begin intervention unless an effort is made to identify the variables contributing to this changing frequency and to incorporate them into the program. Perhaps it is a particular staff member's behavior when interacting with the target patient that (in contradistinction to other staff members) generates this patient's disjointed communication.

Behavior is not capricious; usually reasons can be found as to why it varies. At the very least it is incumbent upon the designer of the behavior modification program to attempt through careful observation to decipher the puzzle. Often the behavior will become stable, if observations are carried out long enough. But the length of time necessary to achieve stability in all cases is impossible to state. Also, no *exact* criteria can be put forth to indicate how long to continue gathering baseline data on unstable behavior after searches for possible causal variables have proven fruitless. Exigencies need to be considered. Obviously, a patient who is severely mutilating himself cannot be observed for a few weeks, days, or perhaps even hours. In cases such as these, measures such as aversive stimulation (see Table VI) or chemotherapy must be used immediately. But this urgency is the exception not the rule, and should not become the prototype for all behavior modification practices m a psychiatric unit. Most often the application of behavioral intervention should be predicated on comprehensive assessment.

Intervention techniques (e.g., positive reinforcement, response-cost) were elucidated in the text and tables of chapter 6. For the behavior modifier several elements overriding the use of these methods are important to reiterate; namely, being systematic, pragmatic, gradual, and thorough. It is the specificity of the approach that is most often abused by novices who attempt to "try it out," or who want to "see if it works." No excuse can be given for this haphazardness.

In chapter 15 we will discuss evaluation in behavior modification. Nevertheless, it is appropriate to mention here that monitoring the patient's behavior through the program is imperative in order to see if the procedures are working in the patient's best interests. In addition we wish to restate that periodic follow-up checks on the desirable improvements that have ensued from the behavioral program should be carried out. The data obtained from these planned measurements may reveal a relapse, necessitating the reintroduction of previously successful techniques.

Behavior modification as a sophisticated technology is a process for helping patients to live more capably. It is *not* a bag of tricks to be applied to seemingly encapsulated problems. Behavior modification must be utilized judiciously. If so it can work for patients and be an invaluable technology for hospital personnel. But if not applied with forethought and precision, it may be useless and perhaps even harmful.

This chapter has suggested that individual procedures can assist in the rehabilitation of psychiatric inpatients by supplementing the hospital's unit-wide program. Some general considerations in the use of individual psychotherapy and behavior modification programs are advanced. Despite their theoretical diversity all forms of psychotherapy should utilize the in-hospital behavior of the patient as the primary data for discussion. This dictum and its implications are explored. The principles of behavior modification programs for individual patients are discussed, emphasizing the need to be thorough, precise, pragmatic, and systematic. These latter qualities are also important when applying another type of individual procedure—the use of psychoactive medications.

Chapter 10

THE USE OF MEDICATIONS
IN A PSYCHIATRIC HOSPITAL

BECAUSE OF THEIR EFFECTIVENESS, psychotropic drugs, such as phenothiazines, anti-depressants, and lithium, have been widely used in the treatment of psychiatric inpatients. Therefore, a hospital staff must possess a thorough knowledge of the use of medication. By stressing the significance of psychopharmacological agents we do not wish to overestimate their importance or devalue the use of other therapeutic methods. Psychotropic drugs are not a panacea for mental illness, and indeed leave a great deal to be desired. What we would suggest is that the role of medication, if properly used, is to alleviate specific target symptoms so that patients can more readily participate in other rehabilitative treatments.

In this chapter we will not attempt to outline the clinical indications, contraindications, and side-effects of medication since these topics are well covered in other books (Klein 1969, Ban 1970, DiMascio 1970b, Detre 1971a). Instead, we will attempt to describe certain aspects of their use which we feel are of particular import to all those who work in a psychiatric hospital. We will present and discuss six guidelines which we have found to be helpful in the utilization of medication in psychiatric units. These are:

1. *All* hospital staff must be familiar with the use of medication.
2. Drugs should only be used when properly indicated; conversely, they should not be withheld when indicated.
3. Staff attitudes towards medication can influence patients' clinical response.
4. The use of psychotropic agents should, as much as possible, become a collaborative venture between the staff and the patient.
5. During hospitalization the staff must try to identify those patients who are currently not taking their medication and actively find ways to prevent this from continuing.
6. During hospitalization the staff must try to identify those patients who are unlikely to take their drugs following discharge and actively discover methods to prevent this from occurring.

GUIDELINE 1: ALL HOSPITAL STAFF MUST BE FAMILIAR WITH THE USE OF MEDICATION

Because the psychiatrist's training specifically provides him with the information necessary to become an expert in the use of medication, this does not imply that everybody else on a hospital staff should be ignorant of clinical psychopharmacology. There are three major reasons why *all* staff, including nurses, aides, recreational therapists, social workers, etc., should be acquainted with the essentials of psychoactive drugs: (a) Patients often ask questions and present doubts about medication to all staff and, therefore, the staff must be able to respond intelligently to these concerns. (b) Because the non-medical staff usually spends more time with the patient than does the psychiatrist, it may often be the first one to detect the onset of side-effects. For example, patients on high doses of lithium carbonate can develop a fine tremor of the fingers which may become grossly apparent only under particular circumstances. This tremor may not be readily discernible in a psychotherapeutic session, but may be more observable to a nurse who sees the patient spilling his coffee, or to an alert recreational therapist who notices him missing keys while playing the piano. Similarly, patients on phenothiazines, especially chlorpromazine (Thorazine), can rapidly develop a painful sunburn and, therefore, precautions to avoid excessive exposure to the sun for these patients should be made by the staff. These observations and precautions cannot be made, however, unless the staff is acquainted with the potential side-effects of medications. (c) Nursing staff, by virtue of its responsibility to dispense drugs, must be aware of potential prescribing errors on the part of the physician.

GUIDELINE 2: DRUGS SHOULD ONLY BE USED WHEN PROPERLY INDI-
INDICATED; CONVERSELY, THEY SHOULD NOT BE WITHHELD
WHEN INDICATED

Medication, like any other treatment method, can be used either to the patient's benefit or to his detriment. Although it can and frequently is prescribed solely as a distancing maneuver, we have been impressed that some hospital personnel, because of their ideological bias, may at times go to the opposite extreme (Fischer 1971). For example, a manic patient was upset that his mother did not come to visit him and began to smash everything in sight despite the staff's efforts to "talk him down." Initially empathetic to the patient, the staff eventually became angry over the patient's destructive activities. As this behavior escalated, the staff was reluctant to use medication, feeling it would have been done out of their own hostile impulses. Finally, the patient, having worked himself into a frenzy, slugged another patient who then required emergency medical attention. After having done this, the assaultive patient became remorseful and fell ino a profound depression. In this example the well-meaning staff might have averted the whole situation by using medication, thus objectively responding to the patient's needs rather than to their own feelings.

Another circumstance where potentially useful drugs might be withheld from a patient is when a therapist tries to demonstrate to the patient, if not himself, that his own skillful psychotherapy is enough. Many studies have demonstrated that appropriate medication facilitates rather than impedes successful individual psychotherapy (Gorham 1964, May 1964, Grinspoon 1967). Even Freud looked forward to a time when the psychological mastery of the unconscious would be assisted by chemical agents (Havens 1970). Thus, medication should be viewed as an ally rather than as an enemy of the psychotherapist.

Finally, we have oftentimes observed the reluctance of hospital psychiatrists to switch to a different class of medication if the one usually preferred fails to achieve the desired effects. For example, a young woman was hospitalized for an acute schizophrenic episode and was placed on adequate doses of phenothiazines. After six weeks, the patient failed to show any discernible improvement, even after the dose was substantially increased. Feeling that nothing more could be accomplished, the staff transferred the patient to a longer-term unit. Upon admission to the second hospital, the patient once again received phenothiazines, but to no avail. At that time psychoanalytic psychotherapy was begun. However, the patient continued in her psychotic state. After four months, a consultant was brought in who suggested switching the patient from phenothiazines to thioxanthenes, another class of anti-psychotic compounds. Within one week the patient showed a dramatic improvement and was discharged soon afterwards. Although we may be suggesting a causal relationship where only a correlative one exists, it is quite possible that the thioxanthenes were responsible for the patient's improvement. If that is so it is highly probable that if the psychiatrist at the first hospital would have tried thioxanthenes after the phenothiazines had failed, the patient would have been spared a protracted hospitalization.

Hospital psychiatrists should not withhold medication from patients just because they are unfamiliar with them, or because they are not the class of drugs usually indicated in the treatment of a particular disorder. In fact the hospital is an ideal setting to institute a succession of drug trials, because it allows for constant observation of the patient's clinical response. The use of medication, like any other treatment modality, should be based on pragmatic rather than theoretical considerations.

In pointing out examples where medication is inappropriately withheld we do not wish to gloss over the need of the psychiatrist to use these potent psychoactive agents judiciously and intelligently. The psychiatrist in *choosing* a drug must be guided by diagnostic considerations, but can only *determine* if the medication is effective when certain maladaptive behaviors are lessened. Therefore, the physician must not only reach a diagnostic decision, but also must be able to identify specific target behaviors in order to have a base line upon which to make a valid clinical judgment about the utility of the medication.

GUIDELINE 3: STAFF ATTITUDES TOWARDS MEDICATION CAN INFLUENCE A PATIENT'S CLINICAL RESPONSE

There is objective evidence to show that patients will accept medication to the degree that the therapist feels it will be beneficial to them (Uhlenhuth 1966, Sarwer-Foner 1970, Irwin 1971). We also may assume that the same result applies to the patient's clinical response. In other words the patient is more likely to obtain symptomatic relief if those prescribing the medication feel that the drug will be helpful. In a hospital setting it is not only the therapist, however, who will influence a patient's attitude toward the drug, but also all those who work with him. Thus, it is not in the patient's best interest to have a psychiatrist advocate the use of a particular drug, while other staff members tell the patient, either explicitly or implicitly, that "medication is a crutch." If the staff differs in its philosophy of medication, this conflict should be ironed out amongst themselves rather than acted upon at the patient's expense. In the meantime it is important that all the staff convey to the patient an optimistic attitude towards the drug's potential effectiveness.[1]

GUIDELINE 4: THE USE OF PSYCHOTROPIC AGENTS SHOULD, AS MUCH AS POSSIBLE, BECOME A COLLABORATIVE VENTURE BETWEEN THE STAFF AND THE PATIENT

Individual, group, and family therapists repeatedly stress the importance of the patient's active participation and collaboration in treatment. And yet, for some reason, this same spirit of cooperation frequently does not prevail around the issue of medication therapy. Traditionally, it has been the doctor who prescribes and the patient who passively receives the psychiatrist's pharmacological gifts (Haven 1963). Although physicians may prefer to shroud themselves in a cloak of unquestioned professional omnipotence, this disguise is not consistent with his approach in other forms of treatment in which the patient's level of competence is encouraged by stressing his active involvement in a joint therapeutic endeavor.

In a sense it is impossible for the patient *not* to be a collaborator in drug treatment, since unless the patient swallows the medication, the drug is unlikely to have an effect. By stating that the patient should be involved in this cooperative venture, we do not mean that the patient ought to determine the type and dosage of medication to be prescribed. Clearly, this is not within the expertise of a vast majority of patients (although an occasional

---

[1] We would like to point out that the three principles already elucidated in this chapter also apply to the use of electro-convulsive therapy (ECT). All hospital staff must have knowledge about ECT since they will be involved in the care of those patients who receive it. Part of any staff education program should be to witness several ECT's as well as to learn its indications, contra-indications, and complications. Like any other treatment, ECT can be used to the patient's benefit or to his detriment. Not to have ECT available, however, is to prevent the patient from acquiring what oftentimes can be a dramatically effective treatment (Fischer 1971). And finally, staff attitudes about ECT are usually quite variable and frequently passionate. Disagreements over ECT should be discussed within the staff and not be thrust upon the patients.

few may be unusually sophisticated in the knowledge of psychoactive agents). Nevertheless, we are suggesting that patients should have some elementary understanding of the drugs they take, the potential side-effects, and the capacity to monitor their own drug related progress (Havens 1963, Lehmann 1970).

Assuming that the hospitalized patient is able to understand what the physician is telling him, the psychiatrist should, before prescribing a drug, provide the patient with some basic information. The patient should know the name of the drug, the symptoms it is being used for, and, unless the patient is unusually suggestive, its common side-effects. They also should be told when it is reasonable to expect a therapeutic response. For example, unless the patient knows that a tricyclic anti-depressant (e.g. Tofranil, Elavil) usually fails to result in a clinical improvement until ten to fourteen days after a therapeutic level has been reached, he may become prematurely discouraged, feeling that the medication has failed to work. Similarly, patients should learn about the periodic use of medication. For example, they should know that taking an extra 25 mg. of an anti-depressant will not result in an instant euphoria, but that small doses of a phenothiazine may provide an immediate calming effect. Furthermore, the abuse and addictive potentials of certain medications should be explained.

Patients should not only know about medication, but also participate meaningfully in the management of their drug treatment by systematically monitoring the target symptoms for which a drug was initially prescribed. For instance, a depressed patient with vegetative symptoms such as weight loss, constipation, and insomnia can daily record changes in these biological variables as well as in his mood. While still in the hospital, a staff member may show the patient how to construct a *symptom chart* (Detre 1971a, p. 89), so that the therapist can receive useful information and the patient can plot his own clinical course. This data keeping can also help the patient to learn about his condition and those symptoms that are likely to indicate a change in his clinical status. In order to encourage patients to correctly begin and main-

tain a symptom chart, it may be useful to provide positive reinforcement such as granting additional privileges. Other patients
on the unit can also help chart one another in order to provide
patients with objective and systematic feedback, while becoming
better and more sophisticated observers themselves. Once again,
positive reinforcement will be useful in rewarding such behavior.

On or even before admission to a hospital we have found it
useful for patients to fill out a form that lists the common side-
effects of psychotropic medication. The KDS-2, a self-administered
questionnaire, is particularly helpful for this purpose (Detre
1971a, p. 93). It lists forty common side-effects of psychotropic
agents, which the patient checks off, if he is currently experiencing them, as well as indicating the degree to which they are both-
ersome. The use of this form illustrates that many symptoms
frequently attributed to medications were present *before* drugs
were actually used. Results of studies with many psychiatric patients show that their so-called "side-effects" decrease rather than
increase after being on medication (e.g. Kupfer 1971a). Unless a
clinician has a base line of symptoms before prescribing a drug, he
will be unable to determine if the "side-effects" are due to the
drug, to the illness, or to both. These forms can also be administered periodically throughout the hospitalization, to systematically
ascertain the development of any new side-effects. In this manner
the patient can keep his therapist up-to-date on possible adverse
effects. This is particularly important, since patients may be reluctant to report some of them unless the therapist specifically in-
quires. For instance, female patients may be hesitant to mention
that they are having a discharge from the breasts unless the staff
deliberately inquiries. Thus, patients can assist in their own therapy by filling out a side-effect check list on a weekly basis.

Afforded the opportunity to do so, patients can also assume
responsibility for their own drug treatment. For example, patients
can go to the nursing station by themselves for medication, rather
than having a nurse search them out. If hospital rules permit,

prior to discharge, patients may be given a number of pills to take on schedule without nursing supervision, as they will be expected to do after leaving the hospital. Patients who "forget" to take their medication can draw up a *drug schedule chart*, listing the name of the medication, its dose and the times of the day it is to be taken. Whenever the patient takes his medication, he indicates this by placing a mark in the appropriate column. By so doing the patient can get in the habit of checking his own reliability. These drug schedule charts can be located in a prominent place in the patient's room so that he can't help but see them. After discharge, this procedure may be continued by having such a chart in a readily noticeable place. These charts can be small enough to fit in a purse or wallet and thereby still serve as a reminder without being overly conspicuous. Both during and following hospitalization, positive reinforcement procedures may be useful in rewarding patients for initiating and maintaining drug schedule charts. Regardless of the methods that are utilized, however, the essential principle is that patients should be encouraged to be an active collaborator in their own drug treatment. To facilitate this the staff should find ways to maximize the patient's sense of responsibility in his own therapy.

GUIDELINE 5: DURING HOSPITALIZATION THE STAFF MUST TRY TO IDENTIFY THOSE PATIENTS WHO ARE CURRENTLY NOT TAKING THEIR MEDICATION AND ACTIVELY FIND WAYS TO PREVENT THIS FROM CONTINUING

Various studies have shown that from five to thirty-two percent of psychiatric inpatients fail to take their medication (F. Forrest 1958, Neve 1958, Hare 1967, Irwin 1971) and that, at least in one investigation (Irwin 1971), sixty-three percent of patients on hospital leave were not taking their prescribed phenothiazines. These facts are particularly disturbing in view of the propensity of patients who discontinue medication on their own to suffer major relapses (F. Forrest 1964, Bernstein 1966, Engelhardt 1967). Therefore, it is important for the staff to be able to identify those patients who are not taking their drugs as prescribed. Although not foolproof, the following practical suggestions in identifying such patients may be useful:

1. *No clinical improvement.* When the staff finds a patient who would be expected to improve with drug therapy but does not, then it is important to ask if the patient is actually ingesting his medication. The absence of clinical improvement may suggest non-cooperation in drug treatment.

2. *Absence of common side-effects.* Many patients who take phenothiazines or anti-depressants will experience a few side-effects, such as dry mouth, constipation, and blurred vision. If none of these is present, it is possible that the patient is not taking the prescribed dose. The absence of these side-effects is not diagnostic of a patient failing to take medication, but is highly suggestive of his doing so.

3. *Ask the patient.* Sometimes it is useful to directly ask the patient if he is taking his drug. We have seen patients go to great lengths to avoid doing so, but if directly asked about it, they will admit to not ingesting them.

4. *Presence of unusual behavior when taking medication.* Any experienced psychiatric nurse knows that some patients will try to "cheek" their medications by holding them in their mouth rather than swallowing them. Patients will then quickly, but calmly, go directly to their room or to the lavatory and dispose of the medication. In order to prevent "cheeking" the nurse should carefully inspect the mouths of those patients who arouse suspicion. Although often useful, this method is not foolproof, since the most experienced patient can outwit even the most experienced nurse. Nevertheless, by checking the patients' mouths, many who are failing to ingest their drugs can be identified. If the patient is still unwilling to take his medication, alternative methods of administration, such as liquid or injectible forms, may be useful.

5. *Urine color tests.* Fairly reliable urine color tests are described by F. Forrest (1957, 1958, 1961) and I. Forrest (1960a, 1960b) that can be an invaluable aid in determining if a particular patient is indeed taking his medication. These simple tests for the presence of phenothiazine metabolites can rapidly assist the staff in determining if the patient is cooperating in the drug treatment.

To remedy a situation where a patient is not taking his prescribed medication, the staff has a number of available strategies. The first thing it can do is simply to ask the patient about his non-drug taking behavior. Although innumerable reasons are given by patients, some of them deserve comment. At times medications are not taken because the patient feels that it is a "crutch" upon which he will become interminably dependent. Closely related to this is the oftentimes expressed belief that the patient is a "slave" to the drugs and that it is the medication and not "him" that is responsible for his improvement. A careful and honest explanation of what drugs can and, more importantly, cannot do, may be helpful in reassuring the patient. It is also useful on occasion to suggest to the patient that true independence and maturity exist when one realistically focuses on one's difficulties and accepts the responsibility for effectively coping with them. More specifically, it can be pointed out that the patient is not a "slave" to the medication; he has the choice to decide whether or not to take his drugs, and that making the choice to do so represents on the part of the patient a decision to maximize his own rehabilitation. On the other hand the patient should also be told that a failure to take his medication represents a decision on his part to risk increasing symptomatology and prolonged hospitalization (Lehmann 1970).

Patients may also fear that taking medication labels them as being "mentally ill." It is important to be alert to such concerns and to explore them thoroughly; for they may serve as not only a resistance to treatment, but also a readily accessible springboard to a discussion of the patient's behavior problems and his feelings regarding them. Other patients may be concerned that taking medication leads to addiction, a loss of sensitivity, a denial of "special insights," or the performance of peculiar behavior. Education and reassurance not only by the staff, but also by other patients, may be of assistance in alleviating many of these concerns.

Sometimes patients are reluctant to take medication because of annoying side-effects. In response to these complaints psychiatrists may overreact in two ways: (a) They may discontinue the medications altogether, or (b) ignore the patient's complaints, labeling them as mere "resistance," and continue the same level of medication. If a patient complains of side-effects we would suggest the following routine:

1. Make sure the medication is properly indicated. If not, discontinue it.

2. If the medication is indicated and has been shown to be useful, look at the patient's base line side-effect checklist to see if the patient had the symptoms prior to being placed on the drug.

3. Many symptoms go away spontaneously within a week or two of medication, or else the patient becomes acclimated to the particular side-effects so that they are no longer troublesome. Thus, make sure that an adequate time has elapsed to allow possible tolerance of side-effects to develop.

4. If this still does not help, consider giving all medication in a single evening dose. Without forfeiting any therapeutic effect, this maneuver has numerous advantages: (a) Patients frequently will experience fewer side-effects throughout the day (Haden 1959, Kramer 1962, Peterson 1963). (b) A single dose at bedtime can often eliminate the need for potentially addictive sleeping pills. (c) It is easier for patients to take a single dose after leaving the hospital than to have to remember to take multiple dosages. (d) Nurses will be able to spend more time with patients and less time dispensing medication, which happens when drugs are given in the traditional three to four times a day basis. Therefore, there is good reason for using a single dose whenever possible, whether the patient has or does not have side-effects (DiMascio 1970a).

5. If a single nighttime dose does not alleviate the uncomfortable side-effects, one should try a drug of a similar class which has a lower incidence for that *particular* side-effect.

6. And finally, if none of the above works, the psychiatrist and the patient have to decide if the "treatment is worse than the disease." In most cases it is not. Perhaps, then, the only recourse is for the patient to learn to live with the consequences of drug treatment.

Other ways to facilitate and encourage the resistant patient to take his medications have been described in Guideline 4. Once again, these involve making the patient an active collaborator in his own drug treatment. At the same time the staff should be alert to the possibility that patients may be more willing to take medication from one staff member than they would be from another. For example, a patient with unusual fears of homosexuality may refuse medications from a young male nurse, but may take them from an older and more maternal staff member. A staff in a reactive hospital environment should be alert to these subtleties.

Sometimes it is essential to the patient's well-being that he receive medication which he is highly resistant to taking. In these situations we have observed staff literally spending hours attempting to coax overtly delusional patients into taking medications, to no avail. Not only is this a waste of valuable staff time, but more importantly, it can result in even further agitation on the part of a patient who feels that the staff is unable to exert sufficient control. In these situations we recommend that after a reasonable time for discussion has elapsed, the nurse in the presence of several other staff members offer the patient a choice between pills and an injection. The patient is given a very brief time to make up his mind. If he persists in his refusal, the nurse no longer discusses the issue, but immediately administers the injection with the assistance of the other staff. At times this kind of necessary confrontation is upsetting to the patient (if not to the staff), and it is, therefore, useful to have a nurse stay with the patient until the latter feels more comfortable.

GUIDELINE 6: DURING HOSPITALIZATION THE STAFF MUST TRY TO
IDENTIFY THOSE PATIENTS WHO ARE UNLIKELY TO TAKE THEIR DRUGS
FOLLOWING DISCHARGE AND ACTIVELY DISCOVER METHODS TO PRE-
VENT THIS OCCURRING

It is one thing for a staff to ensure that a patient takes his medication during hospitalization, but quite another to guarantee that
he will do so following discharge. Therefore, the staff should
attempt to identify those patients who are likely to prematurely
discontinue their drugs after leaving the hospital. For instance,
those patients who have a prior history of discontinuing medication, were resistant or unreliable in taking medication during
hospitalization, or lightly dismissed the significance of their maladaptive behavior could all be included in this high risk category.

It is hoped that by educating the patient and allowing him
to be a collaborator in his own drug treatment, premature cessa-
tion of medication after discharge will not occur. Nevertheless, other
measures may be necessary. Prior to discharge it may help to discuss and to explore with the patient the need for him to remain
on the drug, the possible consequences if he fails to do so, and
some of the common reasons people give to explain why they stop
their medication. Some patients will claim they stop because of
the expense of the medication. Although frequently this is a
rationalization for some other anti-medication feelings, there may
often be a great deal of reality to these complaints; medications
can be expensive (Havens 1968). The therapist can help by selecting less expensive drugs having equally therapeutic effects. Furthermore, staff can direct patients to reliable pharmacists who charge
relatively less for the same medication. Unfortunately, most psychiatrists are oblivious to the economic considerations of taking
medications. Another reason commonly heard for prematurely
discontinuing medication is, "I was feeling so good, I felt I didn't
need them anymore." Prior to discharge the patient should be
warned about utilizing this kind of reasoning in the future.

In addition to these kinds of educational discussions other

types of learning techniques can be helpful in maintaining people on medication following discharge. In order to be effective, these methods should begin during the hospitalization and continue after the patient leaves the unit. For example, the patient may continue to be a collaborator in his treatment by using the *symptom chart* and *drug schedule chart* that he started as an inpatient. Rewards can be offered to the patient contingent upon his properly filling out these forms. Gradually, the rewards and then the charts themselves can be phased out. Hopefully, by this time the patient will have recognized and accepted his need to continue on medications.

Another important factor in determining if the patient will continue on medication following discharge is the attitude of those significant people in his environment. The family, for instance, can either interfere with the staff's efforts or be a valuable ally in the therapeutic program. To ensure that relatives do not denegrate the use of medication to a patient who is in need of them, it is important to ascertain during a family assessment meeting at the outset of the hospitalization the attitudes that each member holds towards medication. The staff may wish to educate the relatives about medication, in much the same way that the patient was taught (Lehmann 1970).

If the patient may be unlikely to take medication following discharge, the family, if cooperative, can be an invaluable help by increasing the likelihood that the patient maintains his drug intake (Ayd 1970). They can provide encouragement, as well as more tangible rewards for the patient in order to reinforce his medication-taking behavior. They can monitor his drug intake and even dispense the pills to him, if need be. Finally, they can inform the therapist, if the patient fails to take his drugs.

Despite efforts at involving the family as an ally of the treatment team, it may be impossible to gain their allegiance or find suitable reinforcers that would assure their cooperation in maintaining the patient on his medication. As a result, alternative strategies should be considered. For example, if the patient trusts the hospital staff, he may return to the treatment facility to pick up his supply of medication. If that is not possible, a nurse could make frequent home visits, where she could guarantee that the patient is taking his medication. In either case it is unnecessary for daily contacts to be made by virtue of the fact that once stabilized on drugs, it is no longer necessary for psychoactive agents to be taken on a daily basis. Ayd (1966) has suggested the use of "drug-free holidays," where patients in collaboration with their therapists can discontinue their medications for two to three days at a time without adverse consequences. By so doing the patient may develop a greater feeling of independence and the staff will be able to reduce its work load (DiMascio 1970a).

And finally, another method for ensuring that patients continue on medication is to use fluphenazine (Prolixin) enanthate or decoanate, which are long-acting injectible phenothiazines. These compounds provide adequate levels of medication for a two to three week period. Although frequently prescribed for patients who are unreliable in taking drugs, they may also be valuable for those who do not wish to be bothered daily by having to remember to take their medication.

In summary the hospital staff should make every effort to identify those patients who will not follow through on their drug treatment and actively seek methods to prevent this from occurring. Failure to do so may result in the hospital becoming, at least for some patients, a permanent dwelling rather than a temporary retreat from the task of daily living.

Chapter 11

ACTIVITIES THERAPY

IN A QUEST for innovative solutions to behavior problems a dazzling array of seemingly diverse treatment modalities has been developed. Occupational therapy, recreational therapy, dance therapy, any-kind-of-therapy-you-can-think-of therapy can be found in many contemporary psychiatric hospitals. Initially confronted with this therapeutic smorgasbord it may be difficult to discern a sensible treatment rationale that is shared by all of these therapies. As a result, for most mental health professionals who are untrained in utilizing these methods, the constructive application of these techniques is poorly understood. Nevertheless, because these numerous techniques can be found in 75% of psychiatric hospitals (Kraus 1972), it is essential that they be based on coherent principles and practiced with reasoned discretion.

Because they share a common theoretical basis, we have chosen to refer collectively to these multiple treatment approaches as "activities therapy." The theoretical principle shared by activities therapy is that the *performance of adaptive activities is incom-*

patible with the practice of maladaptive behaviors. For example, the practice of playing volleyball is incompatible with seclusive behavior. Although this basic principle is easy to acknowledge, oftentimes it can be difficult to implement so that it contributes to the patient's optimal rehabilitation.

FUNCTIONS OF ACTIVITIES PROGRAMS

An effective activities program can provide invaluable diagnostic and therapeutic services in any or all of the following five areas:

1) *Occupational skills.* These include evaluation of and training in marketable and potentially marketable activities, such as academic pursuits, business skills, or household chores.

2) *Daily living skills.* These include the assessment and rehabilitation of behaviors, such as grooming, washing, utilizing public transportation, using a telephone, etc.

3) *Social skills.* These include evaluating and helping to initiate or to increase a patient's conversational abilities as well as his avocational pursuits, such as dancing, playing sports, etc.

4) *Neuro-psychiatric skills.* These include an assessment of and training in behaviors, such as muscular coordination, ability to concentrate, visual acuity, etc.

5) *Emotional skills.* These include evaluating and helping patients to appropriately express or to control strong emotional feelings, such as hostility, affection, jealousy, etc.

Although listed as separate categories, in practice these five types of skills are closely interrelated. Muscular incoordination may affect one's ability to dance; adequate grooming skills may be necessary in order to successfully complete a business transaction. Before attempting to rehabilitate a patient's performance of any of these skills, adequate assessment is necessary.

DIAGNOSTIC FUNCTIONS

At the outset of hospitalization the activities therapist needs to determine which of any of these five types of skills are impaired.

A patient may be able to perform household chores, but unable to express affection to her husband. The specific areas of dysfunction need to be identified. A complete assessment, however, also must determine the skills that will be required by the patient in his post-discharge environment. The ability to grocery shop may be of greater import to a housewife than it would be to a Madison Avenue executive. Thus, a determination of occupational, social, daily living, neuropsychiatric, and emotional skills must be conducted in concert with an assessment of the level and kind of activity the patient will need to possess after leaving the hospital.

In performing such an evaluation, ideally five sources of information should be gathered and integrated in order to determine the patient's activity repertoire. First, an *initial interview* with the patient may be conducted in order to assess his level of skills and to help the patient and the activities therapist become acquainted with one another. Second, a *performance assessment* should be used that enables the therapist to directly observe the patient's ability to accomplish tasks specifically related to his problems. A patient may be assigned some task to perform by himself and others to be carried out within a group setting. In this manner the activities therapist may be able to ascertain the patient's capacity to function in differing situations. Third, a *behavioral survey questionnaire* may be administered to the patient which will yield detailed information about his occupational, social, and daily living skills. An excellent example of this kind of form can be found elsewhere (Mosey 1970, pp. 100-102). Fourth, *reports from other staff members,* such as nurses, psychiatrists, social workers, etc., should be included in the overall assessment of the patient's activity repertoire (Mosey 1970). And finally, *data from significant others* in the patient's environment should be ascertained. For example, a man may state that he was a successful businessman, but a brief conversation with his boss may reveal that he was fired for incompetency. A complete activities assessment, therefore, involves more than simply asking the patient what ails him, but rather requires the use of numerous evaluative techniques. By so doing, a more detailed and hopefully more precise diagnostic evaluation can be ascertained. To merely state that a patient has difficulties in certain skills is inadequate; instead, the specific deficiencies need to be identified. For example, in the case of occupational problems the activities therapist needs to determine at the most general level whether the patient's work capacity is inhibited because of a lack of technical skills, e.g., knowing how to run a machine, or because of maladaptive social habits, e.g., cannot get along with authority figures (Bailey 1968). Each of these distinctions can be subdivided further into more specific behavior difficulties.

At times the data obtained from a multi-dimensional activities assessment may be of value to other members of the treatment team. For instance, certain neurological dysfunctions initially may become apparent during an activities diagnostic evaluation. The activities therapist may be the first to observe symptoms, such as motor incoordination, which in turn can help the physician to reach the proper diagnosis. The major use of an assessment, however, is to provide a basis for an effective activities program.

THERAPEUTIC FUNCTIONS

As was stated earlier, the theoretical treatment rationale for activities therapy is that constructive activity is incompatible with maladaptive behavior. Instead of banging one's head against a wall or sequestering oneself in a bed, patients can be helped by programs designed to enhance their occupational, social, daily living, emotional or neuro-psychiatric skills. An apathetic housewife can clean her room, do her laundry, or make her bed. A socially inept adolescent can learn to dance and to develop conversational skills. An unkempt individual can be taught to bathe, to shave, or to comb his hair. A wife beater may learn to control his violent outbursts by performing vigorous physical exercise. A physically debilitated patient can be started on a gradual program of systematic exercise. By participating in these programs, the patient will be less likely to exhibit, at least simultaneously, maladaptive behaviors.

In designing an activities protocol the therapist needs to identify *specifically* and to implement *gradually* each step of the program. For example, an extremely incapacitated housewife was terrified of shopping. A program was developed and successfully implemented whereby the patient initially stepped outside a mental health center for only a minute. Subsequently, she took a short walk in the direction of a local grocery store. The next day she went to its front door. Eventually, she entered the store and shopped, first with and later without staff accompaniment.

When beginning such a program it is necessary to start at a level where the therapist expects the patient to perform. A common error is to underestimate the patient's performance capacity and to choose a starting point that is considerably below the patient's present level of skill. By continuing to set such low expectations the therapist may constrain patients into conforming to the "sick" role, thereby contravening the activities therapist's traditional emphasis on patients' "healthy" behaviors.

Especially in the beginning stages of treatment, urging someone to develop skills may be inadequate, unless some form of encouragement is provided by way of group pressure or positive reinforcement. For instance, a party-loving college student who was about to be discharged had failed to demonstrate initiative in arranging his academic schedule for the following semester. The unit's activity planning group decided that he would be able to participate in the hospital's weekend social event *if* he submitted a schedule of courses to them before the party. In this example social pressure and positive reinforcement combined to mobilize the patient's adaptive behavior. In some facilities patients receive funds to defray the cost of hospitalization by working to improve the physical plant of the hospital. This type of positive reinforcement is in contrast to the exploitative practice where patients, under the guise of "therapy", maintain the physical facility without financial renumeration. If work therapy is to be prescribed, it should be clear how this activity will be of direct benefit to the patient.

In designing activities that will promote the adaptive skills of patients, the staff must capitalize upon the wide variety of situations provided in a hospital for the performance of these activities. A pianist may give a concert to the patient-staff community; a waitress may wish to work in the cafeteria. In both these examples the patient is provided with a setting in which to practice his skills. This context will approximate the situations he will encounter after leaving the hospital. A psychiatric unit, however, cannot provide all of the potential settings in which one can practice his craft or develop relevant social skills (Wachspress 1965, Haun 1971). Most units are not equipped with airplanes for depressed pilots to fly nor with armies for paranoid generals to lead. Nevertheless, staff can provide situations that can facilitate the rehabilitation of individual patients' behavior problems (Haun 1971). An activities staff can stimulate the pilot's interest in flying by having him discuss his experiences or by allowing him to teach other interested individuals about aircraft. Similarly, the general who may become suspicious when given positions of responsibility could be helped by having him delegate tasks for unitwide projects. Even though every type of occupational setting cannot be provided for within the hospital, it should be remembered that with psychiatric patients more often it is their deficiency of work habits (e.g. punctuality) or maladaptive interpersonal skills (e.g. ability to converse) that prevent them from performing their jobs (Fidler 1963). Thus, it may be helpful to establish situations that require work habits and interpersonal skills that approximate those in one's future employment or social circumstances.

A patient's activities program need not be confined to the hospital setting; it also can be extended to his post-discharge environment. For example, before discharge the patient who has regained housekeeping skills may wish to practice them at home under the gradually decreasing supervision of an activities therapist. Not only will the staff member acquire a first hand knowledge of the patient's future environment, but also the patient will be better equipped to bridge the hospital-community gap.

ABUSES OF ACTIVITIES THERAPY

As is mentioned in the beginning of this chapter, we believe the fundamental principle underlying all forms of activities therapy is that problematic behavior is incompatible with adaptive activities. An application of this concept was elucidated in a nonclinical context by an event that occurred just prior to the outbreak of the Second World War. A journalist asked Hitler why he had his soldiers march so often, to which he responded, "People who march can't think." This statement shows that the aforementioned principle can be used to reach either beneficial or destructive objectives. Presumably, in Hitler's view thinking was a maladaptive activity that was incompatible with what he felt was the constructive behavior of marching. Similarly, in activities therapy it is essential to distinguish between behaviors that will be useful to the patient's ultimate rehabilitation and those antithetical to it. Failure to keep this principle in mind can lead to serious problems.

In order to "cheer up" patients a staff may attempt to transform the unit into an island of utopian virtues, devoid of stress and misfortune. Although at first glance the establishment of a carefree environment may seem to promote adaptive behavior, such endeavors may potentially backfire. If the staff hopes to permanently reinstate the patient into his community, the value systems and social realities within the hospital cannot deviate substantially from those on the outside (D. J. Muller 1971).

Furthermore, it is important to recognize that at times determining the usefulness of certain activities becomes a *relative* matter. There is no doubt, for example, that making pottery in a workshop is incompatible with confining oneself to a bed. A further question that needs to be asked, however, is can other activities be devised that would be equally incompatible with bedrest, but which in addition, would be more helpful to the patient than fashioning pottery? Assuming that the patient will not have access to the necessary materials to make pottery after leaving the hospital, would it be preferable for the patient to be engaged in activities he would enjoy and be able to perform, such as studying, hiking, bicycle riding, etc.? Thus, *sometimes the question is not* if *a particular activity will be helpful, but the* extent *to which it will be helpful* (Fox 1967).

This latter point suggests that when devising activities programs, one must tailor treatment to the needs of the individual patient. To a patient who likes arts and crafts, making a papier-mâché cuckoo may be fun, but to a linguistic professor it may be infantilizing. Because many actvities programs are conducted by individuals who have artistic inclinations, they tend to assume that, since they like making papier-mâché cuckoos, everybody likes making papier-mâché cuckoos. As a result, there is a tendency to call anything we like to do "therapy" simply because it brings *us* pleasure.

On the other hand those who do not have training in activities therapy oftentimes view these treatment methods as a kind of glorified play therapy that "anybody" can do. The skill in being, for example, a competent recreational therapist comes not in being a reliable umpire, but rather in being sensitive to the emotional needs of the patients; the therapist's sensitivity enables patients to participate freely in activities, to learn to cooperate with others, and to gather personal satisfaction from accomplishing one's objectives. Furthermore, competent activities therapists do not create programs just for the sake of entertaining the patients or keeping them busy; hospitalization should not degenerate into a kind of frolicking Mediterranean cruise. Instead, *every* activities program must be geared to the patient's rehabilitation; to do otherwise limits the full therapeutic potential of the psychiatric hospital. If a patient's history reveals that a deficiency in recreational activity has contributed to his impaired functioning, or if fun is demonstrated pragmatically to facilitate a patient's adaptive strivings, then recreational programs are indicated for that patient. We do not subscribe, however, to the belief, as some do (Haun 1971), that having fun for the sake of having fun is a necessary component of a hospital's treatment for all patients. Instead, recreation as well as any other form of activities therapy should be tailored to the particular needs of individual patients.

In closing, a wide diversity of treatment techniques, ranging from occupational training to poetry reading, can be subsumed under the rubric of activities therapy. The potential effectiveness of these therapies lies in the basic assumption that constructive activity is incompatible with maladaptive behavior. It is suggested that a multi-dimensional activities diagnostic procedure will provide an optimal evaluation of a patient's occupational, social, daily living, emotional, and neuro-psychiatric skills. Careful consideration should be given not only to the patient's precise skill impairments, but also to an estimation of those activities the patient will need to perform adequately in his post-discharge environment. In discussing the therapeutic functions of activities programs we have proposed that the staff (a) begin treatment at the level of skills the patient was able to accomplish during his diagnostic assessment, (b) gradually implement programs, (c) provide positive reinforcement for adaptive behaviors, (d) utilize the hospital setting to practice skills he will need to display following discharge, and (e) consider extending the activities program into the patient's post-hospital environment. As with any other form of treatment, activities may be wisely used or greatly abused. Such programs should attempt to provide activities that the patient can realistically expect to participate in following discharge. Hospitalization is too important and too costly an endeavor to be allowed to degenerate into an amusement park experience, unrelated to the difficult struggles confronting psychiatric inpatients as they strive to re-integrate into the community. If a patient is engaged in infantilizing activities, or is exploited by participating in non-remunerative "work therapy," he will not make contact with the rehabilitative potential of the psychiatric hospital. Although it is true that making a belt or mowing the hospital's lawn is incompatible with maladaptive behavior, we would argue that it is of only limited value. Assuming the patient does not have a passion for belt making or lawn mowing it would be relatively more worthwhile for the patient to be involved in activities more directly related to what he actually will be doing following discharge. Thus, it is not enough that activities be merely diversional, they must also be specifically goal-directed.

Of all the specific treatment procedures within a psychiatric hospital, activities therapy tends to focus more upon the adaptive strivings of patients. In one sense activities therapy also seems to differ from many other treatment methods in that it possesses more of a "doing" rather than a "talking" orientation. For these reasons activities therapy would seem to have a unique and important role to play within the psychiatric hospital. Nevertheless, there is no area in hospital psychiatry that has been utilized so extensively, but investigated so minimally. So long as this situation persists, activities will continue to be viewed skeptically by many of those unfamiliar with its merits.

Because activities programs can be conducted as an individual procedure or within the context of a group, this chapter forms a link to the following one. For certainly the collective activity of patients constitutes one type of therapeutic group. There are, of course, many other types of groups which make a significant contribution towards the rehabilitation of psychiatric inpatients.

Chapter 12

GROUP TECHNIQUES

THE HOSPITAL IS AN IDEAL SETTING to utilize group techniques. It is not surprising, therefore, that group psychotherapy originated within a hospital environment. In 1905 at the Johns Hopkins Hospital Dr. Joseph Pratt conducted group discussions with tuberculosis patients, considering the physical and emotional aspects of their illness (Pratt 1906). It was not until after the Second World War, however, that group techniques played a major role in psychiatric treatment. Eventually, these methods became so popular that by the mid-1960's it appeared as if we had truly entered an "age of groups." Therapy groups, encounter groups, unled groups, marathon groups, task groups, and psychodrama were becoming commonplace in American psychiatry. This proliferation of group treatment methods gave rise to an extensive body of theoretical concepts and practical techniques, most of these being developed in outpatient settings. Unfortunately, these same theories and techniques were automatically utilized with psychiatric inpatients. Although useful, we would suggest that models of group treatment based on outpatient experiences do not completely meet the needs of hospitalized individuals. Rather, a theoretical framework specifically designed for the practice of group techniques with psychiatric inpatients needs to be developed.

This chapter will attempt to formulate such a theory and to discuss its practical implications. In no way will we try to thoroughly outline how to conduct group treatment, because other texts provide more complete descriptions (Moreno 1959, Bion 1961, Slavson 1964, Yalom 1970, Solomon 1972) than are possible within the confines of this chapter. Instead, we will present a theoretical model specifically applicable to the practice of group methods within a psychiatric hospital. In so doing we will consider group psychotherapy, staffless-groups, task groups, and psychodrama. A discussion of multiple family groups will be found in the following chapter, while staff sensitivity groups will be examined in chapter 15.

UNIQUE QUALITIES OF HOSPITAL GROUPS

Although they may share many of the same characteristics, inpatient groups sharply differ from outpatient groups. The unique qualities of hospital groups become apparent when considering the *patient population* and the *setting* in which therapy occurs. Generally, hospitalized patients can be distinguished from ambulatory ones in a number of ways. Psychiatric inpatients frequently exhibit greater amounts of behavioral impairment. By dint of being hospitalized, patients often feel they have temporarily abdicated their responsibilities within the community. They may experience a more profound sense of hopelessness and ineffectualness, believing that they are somehow different from the rest of the human race (Harrow 1968, 1969). As a result, inpatients usually have lower levels of self-esteem than do ambulatory patients, particularly those who are chronically institutionalized. The potential for disculturation is more likely to develop with hospitalized individuals. Finally, psychiatric inpatients often tend to display marked dependency upon those delivering treatment.

These patient variables not only interrelate with one another, but also they cannot be separated from characteristics inherent to psychiatric hospital settings.

Any group model practiced with psychiatric inpatients is influenced by the hospital setting in which it occurs. Since most psychiatric hospitals are short or intermediate-term units, inpatient groups generally tend to be of relatively brief duration. Thus, hospital groups tend to have a faster patient turnover and constantly shifting memberships. Although extra-group contacts between patients and staff are the exception in outpatient groups, it is the norm within hospital groups. Since inpatients are living with each other for twenty-four hours a day, events transpiring outside the group frequently become material for group discussions. Conversely, group activities can affect events occurring during the remainder of the day. Unlike those in outpatient groups, hospitalized individuals frequently participate in numerous treatment modalities. Finally, whereas members of outpatient groups can immediately translate what they learn within a group to the outside community, inpatients usually cannot do so because they are in the hospital.

These patient and setting variables need to be considered when attempting to modify group techniques so that they can be more effectively utilized with hospitalized patients. We believe this is true regardless of the specific type of group technique.

GROUP PSYCHOTHERAPY

The most popular current group method within a hospital is group psychotherapy. With this form of therapy four to twelve patients participate under the leadership of one or two staff members. In this context we shall define group psychotherapy as one type of group procedure; its major task is the rehabilitation of individual patient's behavior primarily by means of verbal interchange. Other goals, such as "expanding consciousness," expressing hostility, increasing sensitivity, or promoting fondness are of value *only* insofar as they facilitate the demonstration of adaptive behaviors by the patients.

How this rehabilitation process can be expedited by group psychotherapy is not completely understood. Nevertheless, progress in this area has been made. Numerous models have been formulated, variously stressing insight and transference (Sutherland 1952, Bion 1961, Slavson 1964), transactional behavior (Berne 1966), and interpersonal relations (Bradford 1964, Schein 1965). In treating hospitalized patients, however, we would suggest an *educative model*. Although borrowing from the theoretical concepts previously mentioned, an educative model stresses that group leaders encourage patients to assume the therapeutic tasks of the group. In other words the therapist's primary function is to *train group members* to provide interpersonal feedback, encourage adaptive behavior, offer emotional support, and facilitate the introduction of new members into the group. In a sense the work of treatment becames the major duty of the patients, not the staff.

By educating and encouraging patients to assume therapeutic responsibilities we do not wish to imply that the staff should offer lectures on group psychotherapy. Instead, therapists should utilize situations within the group as the subject matter for the educational process. For example, a woman was describing a fight she had had with her husband. When other patients would interrupt her story by asking questions, she became increasingly hostile. Instead of the therapist immediately interjecting his own interpretations of the situation, a leader who practices an educative model may say, "What does the group think is going on now?" If, as often happens with a novice group, the members fail to reply or plead that they do not know what to do, the therapist should not automatically view this as a "resistance." There is no reason why a beginning group member should know what to do. To "accuse" patients of resisting is neither helpful nor accurate. Instead, the leader could respond with an educative statement like, "Well, one of the ways a group can help Mrs. A (the patient) is by pointing out her current behavior." In this manner the task of making therapeutic comments is delegated to the patients, while the therapists provides them with instructions, directions, and encouragement.

If the group meets often enough, the patients can almost assume full therapeutic responsibility. When this occurs we have heard therapists comment, "The group seems to run itself." This educative model can be so successful that hospitalized patients without prior experience in group psychotherapy have, with a little additional tutoring, become effective group therapists in their own right (Houpt 1972).

If the patients are doing all the work, what then remains for the therapist to do? Essentially, his task consists of setting the boundaries and norms of the group. There are both personal and temporal boundaries. By establishing personal boundaries we mean that it is the task of the therapist to determine which patients should be in the group. By setting temporal boundaries we mean deciding when and for how long the group should convene.

The more difficult problem and the one that reflects the skills of the therapist is that of setting the operational norms of the group. There norms may vary depending upon the preferences of the therapist, but we feel they should include (a) emphasizing the "here and now," (b) focusing on behavior, (c) encouraging open discussion of problems, (d) discouraging inappropriate activity, and (e) stressing the participation of all group members. It is in the ability of leaders to motivate patients to accept and to act upon these norms that the art of being a successful group therapist rests.

Before the patient actually joins the group the therapist should begin to impart these norms. Initially, this can be done by an *orientation* session with the patient. This is especially helpful for hospitalized individuals, because they usually experience a greater degree of anxiety and reluctance to participate than do ambulatory patients. When patients are admitted to a hospital, they do not do so primarily with the intent of participation in group psychotherapy; whereas outpatients usually enter a group because they want to be in one. In order to overcome the resistance and allay the anxieties of hospitalized patients the leaders should orient each patient prior to his first session. This orientation could include an explanation of how groups work, where and when they meet, and what will be expected of the patient. It is also useful to encourage the expression of whatever fantasies and fears the patients may possess, as well as to correct unrealistic expectations or concerns. This orientation can be conducted by therapists or by other patients. Because patients tend to "forget" much of what is told them, a written instruction sheet (see Appendix B) can supplement the verbal orientation.

Although many patients are able to enter group therapy at the outset of hospitalization, others may exhibit behaviors that initially will preclude them from obtaining the benefits of the group. They may be mute, unable to concentrate, excessively hyperactive, or terrified of discussing their problems before other people. Depending on the circumstances, the use of medication, behavior modification techniques, or simple reassurance may be necessary before they can participate. Some therapists may wish to gradually introduce the patient into the group by having him initially observe it through a one way mirror or sit outside the circle. When the patient feels he is ready to participate, he can then join the group as a full-fledged member.

Once the patient enters the group, the therapist needs to consider what kind of communications will facilitate, at least initially, his fullest participation. Although it is difficult to know exactly what these communications should be, a recent study may provide some clues. It was found that hospitalized patients believe that the following four factors were the most helpful in the *initial* stages of a group.

1. *Instillation of Hope.* This refers to a patient's feelings of optimism after having witnessed others in the group improve.

2. *Group Cohesiveness.* This describes a member's sense of being accepted by and attracted to others in the group.

3. *Altruism.* This means a patient finds it helpful to give of

oneself to others.

4. *Universality*. This refers to the satisfying recognition that, contrary to prior belief, one's problems and feelings are not unique, but are shared by others.

It should be noted that these four factors believed to be helpful by psychiatric inpatients were different from those felt to be useful by outpatients (Maxmen 1973a). The latter believed that interpersonal learning, catharsis, group cohesiveness, and insight were the most significant factors (Yalom 1970).

We would suggest, therefore, that at least in the initial stages of the group, the leader should encourage behaviors or communications that stress hopefulness, cohesiveness, altruism, and universality. For instance, if a patient "spontaneously" expresses that he feels better, the leader may respond, "I am glad to hear that. Does the group know how Mr. A accomplished this?" The leader wishes the members not only to identify what the patient did to feel better, but also to support Mr. A's optimistic statement. Some group therapists may feel that this approach is too saccharine and prefer to "puncture his denial." Although hopeful comments may seem phony to the therapist, they, appear, at least in the *eyes of the patients,* to be helpful. Therefore, in the initial stages of a group statements of hopefulness, cohesiveness, altruism, and universality may have greater therapeutic potential than many leaders would expect.

Some may argue that to deliberately emphasize certain factors would interfere with the natural course of the group. We do not agree with this latter position for three reasons. First, instead of leaving things to chance, we feel it is preferable to deliberately arrange situations that will enhance the rehabilitation process. Groups are not inherently therapeutic; they can also be destructive. By purposely stressing certain factors over others therapists may avoid the potentially negative consequences of group interaction. Second, the time-limited nature of psychiatric hospitalization necessitates that the leader become relatively directive in his approach. This facilitates the patients acquiring another group norm, namely, to concentrate on one issue at a time, rather than to flit from subject to subject. And finally, whether or not therapists intend to do so, they cannot help but convey to the members that some factors are more helpful than others.

The frequency that hopefulness, cohesiveness, altruism, and universality need to be stressed depends on the rate at which the group membership changes. Thus, in a short-term hospital where the patient turnover is relatively continuous, these four helpful factors constantly need to be encouraged. On the other hand in long-term facilities, where changes in group membership are infrequent, eventually it would be unnecessary to stress them. Hopefully, after a sufficient duration of time the patients would have developed a sense of hopefulness, cohesiveness, etc.

It is not surprising that these factors are felt to be the most helpful by hospitalized patients who participate in the beginning phases of group psychotherapy. As mentioned previously, psychiatric inpatients, as opposed to outpatients, may have a more profound sense of hopelessness, a deeper feeling of ineffectualness, a lowered self-image, and a belief that they are somehow unique or different from the rest of humanity. In part one can see how these feelings can be attenuated or even eliminated by emphasizing these helpful factors. Furthermore, by training and encouraging patients to assume the responsibility for making useful comments, patients can raise their self-image, feel a sense of accomplishment, decrease their dependency needs, and inhibit the process of disculturation.

In order for patients to undertake a therapeutic role in the group, education and support from the therapist may be insufficient. Additional encouragement in the form of positive reinforcement may be needed to induce patients to assume treatment functions. For example, the concerted pressure of the members can serve as a powerful reinforcer of more useful behavior. This can occur, however, only if the therapist trains, allows, and encourages patients to apply this pressure. Although the use of social pressure can be utilized in all forms of group psychotherapy, hos-

pital staff has the potential to employ additional types of reinforcers. Leaders can reward patients who function as valuable
group members by offering tokens, or by increasing privileges.
Because hospital personnel are able to exert total or at least nearly
total control over a patient's behavior throughout the entire day,
the inpatient group therapist has more opportunity to reinforce
behavior than his outpatient counterpart. By failing to utilize
this advantage, inpatient therapists will be limiting the therapeutic potential of their group.

That rewards can be given during as well as outside the session demonstrates that the effectiveness of group therapy with
psychiatric inpatients can be enhanced if it becomes integrated
with the rest of the hospital program. Leaders should encourage
patients to continue discussing the issues raised in group between
sessions, thereby fully utilizing their time in the hospital. Conversely, events that occur within the hospital but outside the
group can and should be brought into the group for discussion.
This point needs further elaboration.

The majority of therapists believe that the "here and now"
approach is an essential technique for effective group therapy. By
this they mean that therapists and patients alike should eventually
focus the discussion on issues, feelings, and behaviors that are
presently before the group (Sutherland 1952, Yalom 1970). This
is to be contrasted to a "there and then" approach, in which those
participating in the sessions dwell on events that transpired outside the group. The major difficulty with this latter method is
that it is more difficult for leaders and patients to comment on
situations they have been unable to witness. In a hospital setting,
however, many of the extra-group behaviors are witnessed by the
patients and, therefore, can be legitimately and effectively commented upon within the group. Consequently, with psychiatric
inpatients, extra-group comments may be productive, *if* the events
referred to were witnessed by the patients while in the hospital.
We feel this *limited* expansion of the "here and now" approach
helps to integrate the patients' total hospital experience without

doing violence to its fundamental rationale.

STAFFLESS GROUPS

Groups of patients that meet without the presence of staff have been variously called unled meetings (Astrachan 1967), alternate sessions (Wolf 1949, Kadis 1956), and autonomous groups (Hanson 1964, Rothaus 1964). Organizations that are dedicated to the rehabilitation of specific behavior problems also use a form of staffless groups, e.g. Alcoholics Anonymous, Synanon. In recent years peer group therapy has become popular among the more avant-garde of the youth culture. Regardless of how these groups are named, or the goals they possess, their practitioners feel they have considerable therapeutic potential.

Astrachan and his collaborators (1967) have provided us with a systematic evaluation of the nature and utility of staffless groups. They performed their study on Tompkins-I, the intermediate-term/therapeutic community described in chapter 5. They found that in comparison to groups led by staff, there was no statistically significant difference in the degree of interaction, the frequency that patients related content to feeling, and the amount of feedback provided about behavior in the staffless groups. On the other hand in the staffless group there was a statistically greater degree of problem-solving activity. Therefore, this study would suggest that staffless groups function as effectively as those led by hospital personnel, and may even be more helpful in terms of providing practical suggestions to patients.

This latter statement needs amplification and clarification. As the authors have stated, the value of staffless groups may be that they convey to the patients the message that they can be helpful to one another without the presence of professionals. The authors noted that patients in staffless groups imitated behaviors observed in the therapist-led groups in which they participated. Thus, unless the unit's structure provides adequate forums in which patients can learn about what specific topics "should" be discussed, how this can be effectively done and of what the "work" of therapy actually consists, staffless groups can readily flounder into meaningless chit-chat. Given this perspective it is reasonable to believe that staffless groups would have the greatest utility in a psychiatric hospital that provides mechanisms for patients to be able to assume the major role of change agent. That patients in staffless groups exhibit greater problem-solving behavior than those in therapist-led groups may result from a number of factors. Patients in staff-led groups may feel that it would be presumptuous of them to offer guidance, believing that only the therapist has the "real" answers. Psychodynamically influenced leaders may overtly or covertly discourage patients from offering problem-solving statements, feeling that "insight" into unconscious processes or group dynamics may possess a greater significance. And finally, untrained patients may find it easier to provide guidance than to detect subtle interactional phenomena. Thus, the establishment of staffless groups in psychiatric hospitals can be beneficial *if* the unit's structure adequately provides a vehicle for patients to serve as change agents.

TASK GROUPS

Task groups refer to those whose focus is limited to discussions of specific or closely related sets of target behaviors. Groups may be formed which develop basic social and recreational skills, or which attenuate alcoholism, drug abuse, geriatric problems, etc. These groups do not need to be limited to mere discussions, but can involve accomplishing specific tasks; e.g. a geriatric group may plan activities that would be meaningful to them after leaving the hospital.

Any number of staff members could lead these groups. For example, it may be advantageous to have a nurse who has had experience with children conduct a task group of women suffering from a post-partum illness. The hospital may also wish to recruit individuals who are not on the staff to participate in these sessions. A member of Alcoholics Anonymous may be invited to join a discussion group of alcoholics, or a former inpatient may become a permanent member of a discharge planning group. In other words an individual with a specific expertise or personal experience with a particular problem who is not a member of the staff may provide a useful addition to a hospital's task group.

ROLE-PLAYING AND PSYCHODRAMA

If used properly, role-playing and psychodrama are techniques that can serve as effective group procedures. Unfortunately, these two approaches, especially psychodrama, have become rather suspect in the eyes of many psychiatrists because they suggest "acting-out" conflicts rather than talking about them.

Gonen (1971) has defined role-playing as "staging situations which could happen and for which practice can serve as good preparation." He has defined psychodrama as "staging either an actual or a fantasied event in a person's life which is highly emotionally charged and which has never been fully worked through." We will briefly discuss these techniques together, because role-playing can oftentimes evolve into psychodrama.

In role-playing a patient, in collaboration with the staff and other patients, rehearse situations that potentially could become difficult. For example, a patient who may be frightened by the prospect of a job interview may practice having an interview with a surrogate boss. The boss could be played by a staff member, or preferably by another patient who has had trouble being in positions of authority. By rehearsing rather than talking about a problem, patients can sometimes acquire valuable social skills. Video tape feedback may be of special value in this regard (Gonen 1971).

As Moreno (1959, 1966) has pointed out, psychodrama can be group-centered or protagonist-centered. In the former unit-wide difficulties are staged with the intent of clarifying the nature of a problem and hopefully reaching a satisfactory resolution. For example, patients on a long-term unit were distraught over the psychiatric resident therapist's leaving the service. As a result, all therapeutic work appeared to grind to a halt. A psychiatrist played the role of a patient, and a patient played the role of a therapist.

After a while the resident psychiatrist acquired a deeper emotional understanding of how the patients felt about being abandoned, while the patients began to recognize the guilty feelings experienced by the departing psychiatrist. As a result of this group-centered psychodrama, the anxiety level of the unit diminished so that everyone could begin to concentrate again on the task of rehabilitation.

In protagonist-centered psychodrama a single patient acts out a significant problem or conflict in his life. A middle-aged man had felt torn between obeying the orders of his wife and responding to the pleading requests of his mother. Unable to decide between their incompatible demands, the patient turned to alcohol. A psychodrama was staged with two rather domineering females playing the roles of the wife and mother. Eventually, the two women were directed to stand on chairs and peer down at the male patient who was lying on the floor. The women began to shout contradictory orders at him, thereby terrifying the patient. The emotional tension was then accelerated by having the women get down from the chairs and walk over the patient. At this juncture the psychodrama was terminated and the staff and patients discussed what had transpired. From the ensuing conversation it emerged that the man began to realize through the psychodrama that he could not please everybody, and the women became aware of the effects of their domineering behavior. Other patients began to relate how their experiences had resembled what they had observed.

Role-playing and especially psychodrama are not panaceas and can be abused readily by an overzealous staff. Restraint, good judgment, and proper training are necessary qualities for all hospital personnel who wish to stage these group techniques. Nevertheless, these highly emotional and provocative methods can, under the correct circumstances, help patients to recognize those behaviors that interfere with their daily living. As with any other group procedure, patients should be oriented before they participate and may ease their way into psychodrama by first being a member of the audience. This is important in role-playing and especially psychodrama, because they are unusually sophisticated techniques that generally require a considerable degree of spontaneity and abstract thought (Polansky 1969). Thus, if these techniques are to be staged in a short-term hospital, they must be performed frequently so that patients will have the opportunity to learn the methods.

Although role-playing, psychodrama, as well as all of the previously mentioned group modalities primarily have a therapeutic function, their potential use as *evaluative vehicles* should be remembered. By careful observation staff can detect subtle as well as gross behaviors that interfere with the patient's interpersonal relations. Whether a patient relates differently to men or to women, becomes frightened under apparently minimal stress, or responds better to older people than to adolescents, may all be useful data for the treatment team to acquire. Thus, group techniques may provide the patient as well as the staff with important clues as to the nature of an individual's interpersonal relationships.

In summary we have suggested that the practice of group methods may need some modification when utilized with hospitalized individuals. We have outlined some of the important patient and setting variables that would support this contention. Some theoretical as well as technical modifications have been suggested for the practice of group techniques within a psychiatric hospital. Several types of groups have been discussed, emphasizing their treatment and evaluative potential. Nevertheless, in viewing groups one should not forget what is for many people the most important group in their life—the family. And it is to the family that we now turn our attention.

Chapter 13

FAMILY INVOLVEMENT

ACCORDING TO MANY SOCIAL CRITICS, the American family is dying. Some individuals place the blame on "permissive" parents whose loose morality and lack of authority has resulted in a gradual weaking of family ties, while others view the family as an anachronistic institution, failing to meet the needs of those living in a rapidly changing society. Despite the kernels of truth in these diverse perspectives, the family, with all its limitations, continues to be a potent social and psychological force in contemporary life. Nowhere is this so in evidence as when one listens to the histories of hospitalized individuals. For their strongest feelings and attitudes are usually directed toward their families, whether past, present, or future. Thus, to treat a hospitalized patient in the absence of his family is to ignore an essential if not dominant aspect of a patient's existence. The important question is not *if* the family should be involved, but *how* this should be accomplished. Obviously, for some patients family involvement is impossible. Relatives are deceased or totally disinterested, as occurs frequently with many individuals who have been institutionalized for decades. Nevertheless, for the majority of hospitalized patients family participation is a viable and vital component of a treatment program.

The need to involve the family[1] in hospital treatment is derived from two important and frequently occurring facts; namely, patients usually live with their relatives prior to entering the hospital and will most likely return to them following discharge. As a result, it is necessary to involve the family as part of the hospital's program in order to (a) gather information and (b) maximize the patient's chances of optimally maintaining himself within the community after leaving the hospital.

The extent to which families will provide data and assist in aftercare may rest with the staff's ability to encourage the family to become an ally of the treatment team. All too often family members are viewed as intruders or even "enemies" of the patient and those who treat him. Historically, the psychiatrist would speak with the family only under duress, believing that to do so would disrupt the transference. The emergence of theories that speculated about the family's role in the development of psychopathology (e.g., Lidz 1956, Ackerman 1958, Wynne 1958), coupled with the almost exclusive focus in individual therapy on the patient's perception of others, often led to the practice of "blaming" the family for causing the patient's problems. In relating to relatives, however, we believe it is inadvisable, especially at the beginning of hospitalization, to "accuse" them of being responsible for a patient's maladaptive behavior. In the first place it may not be true. In the second place it could unnecessarily accentuate the guilt many family members may already be experiencing. In turn this may prompt them to behave in even more counterproductive and unrealistic ways toward the patient. Finally, by overtly or covertly telling relatives that they are responsible for the patient's condition, we may lead the family, to varying degrees, to resist allying itself with the treatment team.

---

[1] For literary convenience the term "family" will be used synonymously with the word "relative".

Although most families will cooperate with the staff, a few of them will be reluctant to do so. Before accusing these families of being "resistant" to treatment, it is important that the hospital staff examine if they have alienated the relatives in any manner. Because one cannot do family therapy in the absence of the family, we believe that a staff should make every effort, especially at the outset of hospitalization, to ensure that relatives will genuinely cooperate and fully participate in the program. Warmth, empathy, and concern are crucial variables in establishing any kind of therapeutic rapport with a family. In addition to conveying these qualities, it may be useful to specifically tell the family that the staff is "here to help them, not to blame them." If a particular relative is upset, the staff should not hesitate to offer psychotherapy, medication, or even hospitalization (Abroms 1971b).

The task of forging a therapeutic alliance with the family should start at the beginning of hospitalization. At times this may be difficult because relatives may be reluctant or even unwilling to cooperate. They may say that they have nothing to do with a patient's problems and that it is up to the doctors to "fix the patient." Regardless of the feelings underlying these attitudes, it is helpful for the staff to convey to the family the message, "If one member of a family is upset (i.e. the patient), all members of the family are upset." In other words the hospitalization of a close relative is a *moment of crisis*, not only for the patient but also for the entire family. By seeing the relatives on the day of admission, the treatment team can begin to understand the nature of and effectively respond to the family crisis. Also, it is important to immediately involve the family in order to minimize the patient's feelings of having been "dumped" and "abandoned" by his relatives as well as to collect information at the earliest possible moment.

INFORMATION GATHERING

The first major purpose of family involvement is to gather sufficient information from the relatives so as to enable the treatment team to launch a more effective therapeutic program. In order to do so the staff must establish the conditions by which optimal data collection can be obtained. Although the entire subject of family evaluation is beyond the scope of this chapter (see Bodin 1968), it may be helpful to underscore several points. First, it is important that the *entire* family, including children, be involved in the initial assessment. Being less socialized than their parents, children oftentimes provide clues about family skeletons that would not otherwise come to the attention of the staff. For example, the spouse of a depressed patient had told the interviewer that their home life was devoid of strife and he could not imagine why his wife had become ill. Later during the interview his six-year-old son naively asked by his father so often "walks funny." With this clue the staff went on to discover that the husband had been drinking excessively and had at times even become violent. Although parents may object to having their "little ones" exposed to the "ugly" realities of family life, children are not without emotional or observational capacities. They have been exposed to the family's turmoil long before hospitalization, and just about anything they hear during the family interview is usually not new to them. For purposes of initial data gathering we feel that the only reason for excluding children is if they are unable to sit through the evaluation meeting. If not, they should be included for as long as possible.

Interviewing the relatives alone and then together with the patient may yield information not readily obtainable by having only one of these meetings. Hes and Handler (1961) have observed how apparently rational families can act bizarrely when the patient is introduced into the session. Conversely, useful data may emerge only when the relatives meet with the staff in the absence of the patient.

To augment data collection it may be necessary to include significant individuals other than family members in the patient's current social network who have largely contributed to or been greatly affected by the patient's behavior. These may include favored uncles, lovers, employers, neighbors, etc. In a college community roommates and teachers oftentimes serve as a surrogate family and can provide useful information to hospital personnel. At times a visit to the patient's home may reveal information that otherwise would not become apparent in a clinical setting.

In acquiring a comprehensive history from the family and those significant people in the patient's social matrix, we have found it especially useful to be able to answer the following questions:

1. What are the important genetic, developmental and medical factors that have contributed to the patient's current behavior?

2. How does *each* individual in the family define the problem?

3. What are the methods each person has used to cope with these problems?

4. How do family members reinforce the patient's maladaptive behavior?

5. Which relatives are most closely allied and supportive to the patient?

6. What are the positive feelings, common interests, and shared goals of the entire family unit?

7. Who in the patient's environment really makes the final decisions about what will or will not happen in the family?

Although most information gathering will be derived from history taking, observational techniques (Elbert 1964, Bijou 1968, Bodin 1968, Minuchin 1967, LeBow 1972) also can be utilized. Entire families can be given a particular task to accomplish, such as planning the day's activities. The staff can observe how they actually perform this assignment, specifically noting communication patterns, decision making processes, and other forms of behavioral interaction. Psychological tests that may reveal the needs, wishes, feelings, and perceptions of other family members also may supplement the assessment process (Elbert 1964, Bodin 1968). Thus, history taking, direct observation, and family psychological tests can provide the staff with a multidimensional family evaluation. In utilizing any of these family assessment techniques the staff should remember that the *primary* objective is to collect data, rather than to offer treatment. Nevertheless, it is possible that evaluation procedures may be therapeutic for relatives, because family members may learn something about how they function.

As the hospitalization proceeds, it is important to learn how adaptive behaviors by the patient will be greeted by his family. What the staff may view as a positive change in the patient may not coincide with the opinions or the feelings of the relatives. For example, a chronically unemployed 25-year-old single male who finally obtained a job in another city was panic stricken over the prospect of leaving the family nest. The staff's effort to instill a greater sense of autonomy in the patient was thwarted by his over-possessive parents' subtle pleas that their son remain with them. In further discussions with the parents it emerged that having their son at home was becoming a financial burden thereby preventing them from fulfilling a life-long wish of taking a European vacation. The staff proceeded to emphasize to the family that, if their son did accept the job, they would be able to save money and travel. This example illustrates two points. First, the staff and the family may have different goals for the patient which need to be reconciled. Simply ignoring this conflict or saying that the family is "resistant" to change is trivial and inadequate. Second, the staff must help the family discover how they may profit by the patient exhibiting more adaptive behaviors. Just as the patient needs positive reinforcement in order to perform useful activities, the family also needs to be rewarded for encouraging the adaptive strivings of the patient. In the long run this is vital to the patient's capacity to sustain himself in the community following discharge.

In the last illustration the family's less possessive behavior was completely rewarded by the therapist helping the parents to recognize that with their son out of the home they could afford a European vacation. At other times social reinforcers, such as approval from the therapist may encourage the family to redirect their activity vis-à-vis the patient in a more constructive direction. A vital aspect of the ongoing data gathering process is to discover those behaviors of the staff that will potentiate and reward the positive activities of the family.

FAMILY THERAPY IN A PSYCHIATRIC HOSPITAL

The most important reason for involving the family is to sustain and enhance the patient's rehabilitation after discharge. In other words the therapeutic program that is initiated within the hospital should continue following hospitalization, albeit in a somewhat modified form. The staff should teach the family more constructive ways to behave toward the patient and to discover methods that will reward them for so doing. In essence these are the rudiments of any form of family therapy for hospitalized individuals.

One of the advantages of a psychiatric hospital is that it is able to employ a *wide diversity of family treatment methods.* This provides a variety of potentially therapeutic experiences as well as offering the staff the opportunity to determine which approach may be most valuable for the patient in the post-discharge phase of treatment. Another unique quality of the inpatient use of family therapies is that the staff can *control the patient's access to relatives.* Unlike ambulatory care, the family's contact with the patient can be monitored, regulated, and even restricted by the hospital staff. At times this may be necessary for therapy to eventually succeed. For example, a patient was hospitalized for physically attacking his father with whom he had had long standing conflicts. Before he was admitted, bi-weekly outpatient therapy had failed to alleviate the situation. These stormy sessions were oftentimes followed by even more intense disputes after leaving the psychiatrist's office. In order to defuse the explosive situation, the patient, after nearly stabbing his father, was hospitalized. On the day following the admission the family visited, an argument ensued, and within ten minutes the patient assaulted his father. At this juncture, father's visits were stopped and intensive work was begun *separately* with the patient and his father. After some tentative gains were made, the father was allowed to see his son under staff supervision for only five minutes. The duration of these visits was gradually increased contingent upon the patient and his father demonstrating appropriate self-control. The successful resolution of this family conflict would probably not have been possible without the hospital staff's capacity to control the father's access to his son.

As was mentioned earlier, another important aspect of hospital family treatment is that the admission of a patient nearly always results from or contributes to a family crisis. This may require that the staff be direct and decisive, while at the same time empathetic and reassuring. The treatment team should appropriately respond to the immediate needs of the patient and his relatives.

By family therapy we do not mean the utilization of any particular treatment model, but rather the application of numerous methods that are pragmatically chosen on the basis of their potential effectiveness. Although a complete discussion of the multiplicity of available techniques would be too extensive for a single chapter, those of particular utility in a psychiatric hospital deserve comment.

Nuclear Family Therapy

By nuclear family therapy (NFT) we mean a broad group of treatment techniques that are utilized by the patient and his immediate family (e.g. spouse, children, parents, siblings). This is to be distinguished from treatment methods that include individuals beyond the nuclear family (e.g. multiple family therapy, network therapy, etc.). As numerous publications would indicate (e.g. Beels 1969, Erickson 1972, Sager 1972b), the principles underlying the practice of NFT are almost as numerous as those who write about them. If a hospital family therapist is to be able to select pragmatically from a wide diversity of treatment methods, it is important that he be familiar with them even if he does not completely subscribe to their premises.

Unfortunately, the vast majority of these theories automatically tend to assume that the patient's maladaptive activity is *solely* the result of the family's pathological behavior. As a result, they have a proclivity to overlook the possibility that the patient's behavior may have influenced the family to act in a counterproductive manner. We would suggest that, to a greater or lesser degree, both of these situations usually exist simultaneously within the same family unit. The extent to which either of these possibilities is present should determine the general approach of NFT. Before commencing family treatment it is important for the staff to determine the degree to which the relatives' behavior is primarily the *cause* or the *result* of the patient's particular problem. Although with long-standing problems this determination is difficult to recognize, in most cases it can be ascertained by careful family assessment.

Patient-Centered Family Treatment is indicated when the patient's aberrant behavior has resulted in maladaptive or inadequate responses from the rest of the family. For example, a 16-year-old girl was admitted for severe weight loss and was diagnosed as having anorexia nervosa. During the initial contact with the entire family the social worker observed the parents frantically urging the patient to eat. The more they pushed, the more stubborn she became. Initially, the social worker began to think "No wonder the girl doesn't eat!" After gathering further history, however, it became apparent that prior to the patient's dramatic weight loss the family was a reasonably normal one. It was only after she began to starve herself that the parents became desperate. In this instance the task of family therapy was to help the family learn and practice more constructive ways of relating to their daughter. They were instructed to stop pestering her about food and to praise her positive actions. Although certain historical data suggested that mother's overzealous admiration of movie stars *may* have initially influenced the patient to lose weight, this possibility only was explored later in the treatment. The first and primary task was to focus on the family's frantic response to the patient. Thus, in this form of NFT the behavior of the parents is primarily treated as a consequence of the patient's aberrant activity.

Family-Centered Family Treatment is indicated when family conflicts have primarily been responsible for the patient's disturbed behavior. For example, a 17-year-old boy had overdosed on barbiturates which he had stolen from his mother. When the family was seen, it became obvious that his parents had been fighting over the last several months, leading to his mother's increasing abuse of drugs. It was hypothesized that among other things the patient's overdose was primarily perceived by him as a way of escaping from his parents' constant feuds. A family-centered approach was initiated to focus attention on how the difficulties between the parents had resulted in a near tragedy. At first the parents met with the social worker without the presence of their son in order to emphasize the point that the parents had to examine their own behavior. Role-playing and video tape feedback supplemented the exploration of parental conflicts. Once these problems began to resolve, the patient and his psychiatrist were introduced into the sessions so that the parents could demonstrate to their son their changed behavior and the entire family unit could discuss their mutual conflicts and shared aspirations. Thus, in this type of nuclear family therapy the behavior of the patient is primarily viewed as a consequence of the family's interpersonal problems.

It is preferable to view these approaches to NFT as existing on a continuum, rather than being distinct entities. Therefore, on one end of the spectrum is patient-centered family therapy where the task is to aid the parents in finding better coping mechanisms, while on the other end of the spectrum is family-centered therapy where the task is to modify behaviors within the family system that are largely responsible for the patient's condition. Because these two approaches exist on a continuum, the staff must determine the *degree* to which therapy should be patient- or family-centered. Thus, at least *theoretically,* one can speak of family therapy being 25% patient-centered, 75% patient-centered, etc.

Of course in the estimation of the staff, these percentages may change as new information arises during the course of family treatment. In any case what is of utmost importance is that the relatives become actively involved in the hospital's rehabilitation program.

Multiple Family Group Therapy

By its very nature the psychiatric hospital is an ideal setting in which to utilize multiple family group therapy (MFGT). First conducted by Detre in 1960 (Detre 1961b), MFGT is a family treatment technique in which four to seven families meet together in the presence of two therapists in order to discuss mutual problems, provide feedback to one another, and hopefully diminish maladaptive behaviors. Although the theory and practice of MFGT has been described elsewhere (Hes 1961, Laquer 1964, Levin 1966, K. Berman 1972, Tucker 1972), it may be useful to discuss its potential utility for families of hospitalized patients.

Its major advantage is that it can provide certain experiences that cannot readily be derived from nuclear family therapy alone. These include:

1. *Universality.* Because the admission of a patient to a psychiatric hospital is a family crisis, relatives oftentimes feel that they are the only ones in the world that are experiencing difficulties. By participating in MFGT they can discover that they are indeed not alone, but share problems with many others (Norton 1963).

2. *Socialization and Support.* Like patients, family members frequently need to develop and practice their social skills, as well as to be provided with honest, yet empathetic support from those outside the family (Hes 1961, Levin 1966). Universality, socialization, and support allow for the development of the remaining advantages listed below.

3. *Catharsis.* "It felt good to get things off my chest" seems to be a comment heard more often after MFGT sessions than after NFT meetings (Tucker 1972). Catharsis may be inhibited in the

latter type of meeting because the relatives feel that they will be "judged" by the staff. In MFGT, however, where the staff patient ratio is oftentimes 2 to 40, the therapist's presence appears less ominous. As a result it may be easier for family members to discharge strong emotions in front of one's supposedly more sympathetic peers (Curray 1965, J. Lewis 1965, Harrow 1967, K. Berman 1972).

4. *Problem Solving.* Practical solutions to problems offered by families who have shared similar experiences can at times have greater meaning and utility than those offered by staff in NFT (Harrow 1967). If these sessions include families that have recently had a patient discharged from the hospital, everybody can learn first hand about the practical difficulties in readjusting to community life. Frequently, these problems are as great for the family as they are for the patient.

5. *Instillation of Hope.* It is one thing for a family to receive optimistic reassurance from the staff, but quite another to hear it directly from other families who have shared similar experiences. This is possible because MFGT can include families who are in all stages of hospitalization, as well as those who have had a family member recently discharged (Hes 1961).

6. *Inter-Family Learning.* Relatives can provide feedback about each other's behaviors based upon their own experiences. Also, they can learn about how other families have attempted to cope with similar problems. One of the unique advantages of MFGT is that sometimes relatives will be more receptive to listening to the point of view of another patient who is not a member of their own family. Once having acquired this understanding, frequently they are better equipped to "listen" to the patient in their own family. And finally, relatives can witness their own behavior reflected in the actions of others (Hes 1961, Harrow 1967, K. Berman 1972).

7. *Facilitate Other Meaningful Inter-Patient Contacts.* In many psychiatric hospitals patients are encouraged to provide feedback to one another about their particular problems. Frequently, these

problems involve other family members, which are difficult to comment upon meaningfully, since the other patients have only casually, if at all, met the relatives. Therefore, remarks based on little first-hand knowledge, such as, "You got to stand up to your husband," are oftentimes made to patients without any direct understanding of what "standing up to husband" really entails. In MFGT patients are afforded the opportunity to witness directly the behavior of members of other families, and thereby acquire a fuller understanding of the relatives of their fellow patients. In this manner they can provide more accurate feedback to one another (Tucker 1972). For example, in traditional group therapy Mrs. A kept telling the other patients that her husband would never talk to her; the other patients sympathized with Mrs. A's dilemma. Increasingly Mrs. A languished in self-pity. When the same group of patients actually met her husband in MFGT, it became apparent that Mr. A had tried consistently to talk to his wife, but to no avail. In the next group therapy meeting the patients changed their approach to Mrs. A and confronted her about her non-responsiveness to her husband. This latter and more useful discussion could not have transpired, however, unless the patients had heard Mr. A's side of the story.

8. *Data Source*. Although nuclear family therapy can provide information about intra-family behavior, it may be an inadequate source of data for determining how relatives relate to those outside their own immediate families (Hes 1961, Tucker 1972). Thus, while MFGT does not eliminate the need for NFT, the former can offer many therapeutic and evaluative functions that the latter is less able to provide.

Many authors have attested to the benefits of multiple family group treatment in a hospital setting. Laquer *et al* (1964) have reported that 67% of the participating families believed that increased communication and understanding resulted from this experience; 21% were doubtful about its value; while 12% disliked the therapy. With the same client sample the authors felt that 46% of the families demonstrated marked improvement,

32% showed some improvement, and the remainder were unimproved. Levin (1966) found a very high patient and relative attendance in a voluntary multiple family group. He felt there was considerably more interaction in the family group than in the traditional group therapy setting. Hes and Handler (1961) contrasted groups of only relatives (relative groups) with those of relatives with patients (MFGT). They observed that, while the tenor of the relatives group was social and supportive, the tensions in the multiple family group often became unbearable with many previously unrecognized neurotic and psychotic symptoms emerging from family members. Lewis and Glasser (1965) have had similar results in a day care treatment center.

In a more systematic investigation Harrow *et al* (1967) contrasted MFGT with conventional group therapy in a hospital setting. They found the addition of family members facilitated rather than inhibited the therapeutic process. They discovered that multiple family groups had significantly more verbal interactions and were less depressed in tone. Furthermore, there were more comments in which one member would describe another's emotional state, attitudes or behavior than there were in traditional group therapy. These results have been supported by K. Berman (1972) who established MFGT with recently discharged Veterans Administration patients. After 12 months none of these patients had been readmitted whereas formerly 30% to 40% of patients with similar characteristics had reentered the hospital. Collectively, this data would suggest that MFGT not only is well equipped to actually deal with emotionally loaded topics, but also may be useful in maintaining patients within the community.

FAMILY PARTICIPATION IN AFTERCARE PLANNING

In conducting any form of family treatment in a hospital setting it is easy to forget that its prime function is to alter the patient's discharge environment so that he may permanently function within the community at his highest possible level. In so doing it is important that the family therapist (a) specify the maladaptive behaviors of either the relatives, the patient, or both, (b) determine useful alternative activities, and (c) help the patient or his family redirect their previous patterns of behaviors and reinforcers in order to produce more constructive ways of interacting (Liberman 1970, Patterson 1970b).

For example, a 44-year-old female biology teacher was admitted for a total inability to function at home or at school. Prior to hospitalization her husband would frequently leave his job early in order to maintain the household and to offer sympathy and support to his wife. Despite his efforts the patient increasingly became apathetic. During the initial stages of hospitalization it became apparent that the patient, who was in menopause, felt that her worth as a female was irreversibly declining. She believed she had nothing to offer her husband and was afraid of losing his love. Feeling increasingly frustrated and unable to share anything with his wife, the husband began to wonder if indeed his wife's self-perception was accurate. The family therapist speculated that the patient's apathetic behavior was the only way the patient had discovered that would elicit her husband's affection. In order to modify the target behaviors (i.e., poor housekeeping, feeling that patient could not offer anything to husband, and general apathy) a treatment plan was devised to alter these maladaptive activities. Husband was told to respond with affection only for positive behaviors emitted by the patient; apathetic behaviors were to be ignored. Although this was difficult for the husband, he was able to maintain this stance because the staff and those who attended MFGT provided him with support for these activities (i.e., social reinforcement). In the meantime the patient was given household-like tasks to perform on the unit. Her reward for successfully accomplishing these duties was affection from the husband. As her self-esteem began to rise, she was given the task of tutoring biology to the adolescent patients on the unit. For such activity the husband again would offer praise to his wife. As they began to discuss her teaching, husband spontaneously expressed an interest in learning some biology himself. With the encouragement of the staff the patient began teaching fundamental biology to her husband who continued to provide social reinforcement for his wife. This program persisted after discharge with gratifying and enduring results. In this example the treatment team identified the symptomatic behaviors, determined useful alternative activities, and modified the system of social reinforcement within the family. It should also be noted that the staff utilized the hospital milieu in order to help the patient practice behaviors that would be useful after discharge.

In this case the husband's genuine concern facilitated the efforts of the staff. But what about the situation where the patients have been in the hospital for many years without any apparent interest on the part of the family? Many patients, especially those in state facilities, have languished there for 15 or more years without having any visitors. In these circumstances the possibility of discharge and successful adaptation to community life oftentimes seems impossible. To remedy the situation O'Brien and Azrin (1973) have tried what is called "interaction-priming." They took three patients who had little or no contact with their families for between 14 and 30 years. A formal invitation was sent to the relatives asking them to visit the patient in the hospital. Nobody came. Then a contract was established with the family which specified that a member of the treatment team would accompany the patient to the relative's home. During the visit the staff member would say every 15 minutes "It's time to go now", thereby allowing the family to request or not request the patient to stay. In this way family members were more receptive to the program because they did not feel put upon by the staff or by the patient. During the visits the patient would perform *constructive* duties around the home which resulted in praise from the relatives. After nine weeks, two of the three patients were successfully discharged to their families. Bi-monthly follow-up visits by the staff revealed that the patients were able to successfully maintain themselves within the community for at least a two year period. The third patient, who had been in the hospital for almost 14 years, remained institutionalized because of financial and space limitations in the family's home. Although a job placement fell through, vocational training was in progress. This study also suggests that hospital personnel at times may need to make home visits, if successful aftercare is to be launched.

In many facilities patients spend weekend passes with their families in order to practice newly acquired behaviors and thereby to smooth the transition from hospital to home. Staff accompaniment may be invaluable in maximizing the success of such a visit, as well as reporting back to other hospital personnel information regarding what transpired during the pass. At other times such staff accompaniment is neither desirable nor feasible. Instead, the staff may wish to conduct a kind of MFGT session on Sunday evening. This "pass meeting" includes only those patients and family members who were involved in the patients' weekend activities. The meeting limits its discussion to difficulties that may have arisen during the pass.

In sum the family or those significant people in the patient's social matrix need to be involved in the hospital's treatment program. This is necessary for two reasons, namely, information gathering and preparation for aftercare. In order to accomplish these tasks the treatment team should try to induce family members to become its ally. The staff should be responsive to the relatives and recognize that the admission of the patient represents an important crisis in the life of a family. Hospital family therapists have the advantage over their outpatient counterparts in being able to control the frequency and setting of patient-relative interactions, as well as being able to provide a multiplicity of treatment techniques. In utilizing these methods the staff must decide the extent to which family treatment should be patient-centered or family-centered. The potential value of MFGT is discussed, mentioning its specific utility in a psychiatric hospital. And finally, it was noted that family therapy of hospitalized patients should be directed toward modifying the behavior of the patient and his relatives. Hopefully, this will ensure the patient's successful and enduring stay within the community. To do so the treatment program started within the hospital should continue, though in a modified form, following discharge. The importance of successful aftercare planning cannot be underestimated, and will be discussed in the next chapter.

Chapter 14

PLANNING FOR AFTERCARE

FOR MOST PATIENTS *the* major function of psychiatric hospitalization should be preparing for aftercare. This seemingly dogmatic statement is valid, if one believes that the ultimate goal of hospitalization is the permanent re-integration of the patient into the community. It is easy for staff to overlook this perspective by focusing excessively upon particular treatment procedures or by tenaciously attempting to have the patient adjust to life inside rather than outside the hospital. A staff that becomes distracted in these ways may neglect to adequately attend to the primary task of hospitalization, aftercare preparation. Thus, the significance of aftercare planning cannot be overestimated; indeed, *every* principle and technique that has been discussed up to this point is worthwhile *only* to the extent that it sets the stage for successful post-hospital functioning. Aftercare preparations must be an integral part of the total hospital program.

We shall define aftercare procedures as those techniques initiated within the hospital that attempt to consolidate the gains achieved during hospitalization and to maintain them for and to extend them to the outside environment. Hopefully, these techniques will eventually enable the patient to become a permanent, useful, and relatively contented member of society. The technology of aftercare seeks not the "happy ending" *per se*, as much as it attempts to maximize its eventual probability. In this chapter we will present some principles and methods for hospital practitioners to consider when striving towards this objective. Although our knowledge of the theory and techniques of aftercare preparations is limited, several principles are worth considering.

PRINCIPLES OF AFTERCARE PLANNING

Aftercare planning can be divided arbitrarily into two interrelated tasks. The first one is concerned with preparing the patient for his successful adjustment to community life by altering the maladaptive behaviors of the patient, as well as those in his discharge environment (e.g. home, school, work). It is our belief that this task is the major function of aftercare planning, since it is in the community that the patient will spend the vast majority of his time following discharge. The second task is to ensure that the patient receives optimal professional care after leaving the hospital. Although formal outpatient therapy is vital to the overall rehabilitation of previously hospitalized individuals, it cannot be viewed as a substitute for carefully attending to the total life situation facing the soon to be discharged patient.

Environmental Issues for the Discharged Patient

For the most part members of society are expected to work, to communicate, to socialize, to demonstrate acceptable grooming habits, and to have a minimum of inappropriate behaviors. We recognize that not all individuals in every subculture share or even emphasize the same standards of conduct. Nevertheless, in order for a former psychiatric inpatient to maintain himself within any community or subculture, he generally needs to be able to work at some task, to converse effectively, etc. Thus, the staff must ensure that prior to discharge *the patient performs and is capable of sustaining behaviors that will be compatible with the expectations of his particular subculture.* This includes not only the reduction of problem behaviors, but also the acquisition of skills that will be useful in his social matrix. Consequently, in aftercare planning it is crucial to find ways by which the patient can add to rather than detract from the lives of those with whom he will live. Will he serve as an asset rather than a liability, enliven in contrast to impede, support as opposed to burden those people he will most frequently encounter? All too often hospitalization strives only to render the patient tolerable to his family, rather than to focus on how he may actually contribute to it. In the previous chapter we referred to a study in which institutionalized patients who had not received a visitor for between 14 and 30 years were successfully discharged to their homes. An important element in this investigation was that patients were taught to perform useful activities, such as house cleaning, which seemingly increased their family's desire to have the patient return to live with them (O'Brien 1973). Relatives can accept a recently discharged patient under one of two conditions: out of a sense of duty, or because the patient has something constructive to offer them. It is the latter that most enhances the patient's chances for a durable residence within the community. Not only should the patient behave in ways that will be acceptable to those with whom he lives, but also *he must be taught about what he may realistically expect to encounter outside the hospital.* He needs to anticipate and to learn new ways of coping with the typical, although not always desirable, behavior patterns of those in his future environment. For example, after overdosing on barbiturates, a 15-year-old boy was hospitalized. His suicide attempt had followed an altercation with his frequently intoxicated father who, despite the staff's diligent efforts, continued to drink excessively. The focus of aftercare planning involved teaching the boy methods of dealing with his father's alcohol-induced rages. He was taught to stay out of his father's way when he was drunk by either going to his room or visiting a friend. Although hardly an ideal solution, it was clearly preferable to suicide. There are, of course, many other types of difficulties a patient may encounter and need to contend with after leaving the hospital. The problems of reconstructing one's life, overcoming loneliness, and contending with the sense of being either stigmatized or patronized by those in the environment (Bachman 1971) are important issues to be explored prior to discharge. Although these potential difficulties can be exaggerated by both staff and patients (Gove 1973), nevertheless, it is important for patients to anticipate and to learn ways of coping with these types of problems.

Assuring that the patient will be *responsive to the rewards and recriminations society gives to its members* also bears upon his eventually successful adjustment; hence, it may become a major goal of aftercare planning. It is clear that individuals outside a hospital do not always behave like staff do within the hospital. If staff consistently attend, for example, to the patient's constructive activities *throughout* his entire stay, they may be perpetuating a schism between what they do and what society typically does. Towards the end of the patient's hospitalization, therefore, staff may wish to interject a planned inconsistency into their rewarding procedures. At this point all of the patient's adaptive strivings should not result in approval—some should, others should not. In many respects this will assist the patient in becoming acclimated to society's typical patterns of rewarding useful behavior. On the outside individuals are not praised for every constructive activity they perform. The hospital may not be able to resemble the community in every fashion, but it can attempt to do so, at least in some important ways.

One of the most significant areas in aftercare planning is *environmental restructuring*. The aim of this endeavor is to make the patient's post-hospital environment more reactive to his adaptive behaviors. Efforts to restructure the patient's home life should actually begin at the time of admission, when the patient's family and those significant people in his social matrix are first interviewed by the staff. Part of this initial evaluation would include assessing the family's typical patterns of interaction in order to ascertain the extent to which the family aggravates or ameliorates the patient's condition. Although valuable, this first impression may present a distorted picture of family life, because when relatives are first seen it is usually in a moment of crisis, and family members may act in ways that are not indicative of their usual behavior patterns. As hospitalization proceeds and the family crisis subsides, the information from the initial evaluation may need to be augmented and possibly re-interpreted. When a family's behaviors begin to stabilize, it is reasonable to assume that such activity is reflective of its typical state. At this point the staff can begin to modify the family's interactional patterns by any of the methods outlined in the previous chapter. The hospital staff should strive to alter distorted communication, ineffective reward and punishment practices, and unreasonable expectations of the patient. Furthermore, they may wish to educate the family about the patient's problem behaviors, the potential danger signals of an impending decompensation, and the proper use of psychotropic medication. The staff's efforts at restructuring the patient's environment must not only transpire within the hospital, but also within his discharge environment.

As discharge approaches, specific plans may be made to have the *family continue and expand the hospital program within the patient's outside environment.* For example, a very apathetic middle aged man would do nothing but sit around his brother's home, blankly staring at the four walls of his bedroom. Frustrated in all attempts to mobilize the patient, his brother had the patient admitted to the hospital. A behavior modification program instituted within the hospital rewarded the patient's socialization activity with permission to sit in his room. Although the patient improved while on the unit, it seemed necessary to extend the program to the patient's discharge environment, if these gains were to be sustained. As a result, the treatment team trained the patient's brother and sister-in-law to administer a behavior modification program within their home. Although considerably more complicated, essentially, the patient would be allowed to engage in activities he desired contingent upon his performance of useful household chores. After discharge the staff continued to meet with the relatives and the patient at bi-weekly intervals in order to correct any "bugs" in the system, to evaluate the program, and to provide social reinforcement for the family. Thus, a treatment plan begun in the hospital was extended to the outside environment. Another example of this principle is illustrated in the case of a woman who was brought to the hospital following uncontrolled episodes of "histrionic" behavior. The history revealed that she had been chronically dissatisfied with her husband and became involved with another man. When she was suddenly jilted by this other man, she began to cry incessantly, to throw things, and to scream at everybody in sight. Once she calmed down the patient explained that she "didn't love her husband," and, therefore, had tried to have the affair. Upon direct questioning she was unable to specify what exactly was lacking in her marriage. Unable to respond to his wife's ill-defined complaints, the husband increasingly became frustrated and threatened divorce. In conjoint therapy the couple spoke in vague generalities about their relationship, thereby preventing any appreciable progress. At this juncture the staff decided to have the couple negotiate a behavioral contract. She agreed to clean the house and to cook the meals in exchange for his spending 20 minutes talking with her daily and taking the family out to dinner once a week. Both agreed not to argue in front of the children. This contract was first tried out during a weekend pass from the hospital. It worked. After discharge, the couple continued to meet with the treatment team in order to assess their progress and to expand the terms of the agreement. Gaining pride in their own accomplishments, the husband and wife eventually developed a greater sense of affection for one another. Both of these examples illustrate an important principle in aftercare planning; namely, *that programs begun inside the hospital should be extended into the patient's home environment with the help of those individuals with whom the patient will live.*

Attempts at environmental restructuring may be facilitated by having the treatment team make *home visits* following discharge. In so doing they can monitor activities in the home and thereby avert any incipient difficulties. Frequently, regular hospital personnel do not have the time to devote to such activities. As an alternative solution, the unit may wish to employ a "cadre" of paraprofessionals who, although not part of the daily hospital routine, would be intimately aware of the patient's problems, treatment, and progress, and thus could make useful home visits. This could help in smoothing the transition from hospital to community life.

An overriding principle in planning for this transition is *gradualness*. Relatives, for example, should not be expected to *suddenly* alter their behavior as soon as the patient is released. Similarly, discharge plans should not be made on the final day of hospitalization. Instead, preparation for the patient's return to the community needs to begin early in the hospitalization. Furthermore, patients gradually should experience living outside the unit *before* they are discharged. For example, a patient may initially go outside the unit with another patient for an hour, and then spend two hours at dinner with his family, followed by a succession of one- and then two-day passes at home.

Prior to discharge it may be necessary for some patients to have a *completely structured day* awaiting them on the outside. All too often we have seen patients go home "for a rest" rather than to maintain the high level of functioning they exhibited on the unit. A "rest" may be necessary for convalescing surgical patients, but it can be potentially regressive for discharged psychiatric patients. In order for the patient to have a completely structured day when he returns home, it is oftentimes helpful to work out a detailed schedule of future outside activities while the patient is still in the hospital. Whether the day will consist of academic, occupational, or recreational pursuits, these endeavors gradually should be tried out prior to leaving the unit in order to discover any remaining deficiencies in the patient's repertoire of adaptive skills.

This information can be ascertained by a number of different types of meetings or programs. As previously mentioned, home visits may be of exceptional value in this regard. *Discharge planning groups* consisting of soon to be released patients can meet in order to specifically focus on problems they will encounter after leaving the hospital. *Pass meetings* can be held for those patients and their families who have had a patient visit for the weekend. Each individual should report his version of what transpired over the weekend, and the group can focus upon specific aftercare issues. In the previous chapter we also mentioned how families of recently discharged patients may return for multiple family group therapy sessions in order to discuss any problems insufficiently dealt with during the hospitalization, as well as to continually reinforce the adaptive strivings of the patient and his family. The point is that careful attention should be directed to aftercare planning, and that preparation for discharge should be a gradual rather than an abrupt process.

Before actually leaving the hospital it is important for the staff to discuss with the patient those specific issues which will need his attention following discharge. One of the authors has found it helpful to have patients specify in writing a detailed rank order of problems to be dealt with after leaving the hospital. This not only assists the patient in identifying what needs to be accomplished, but also conveys the message that hospitalization is only one stage in his overall rehabilitation. At the same time potential danger signals of incipient decompensations may be discussed so that the patient can possibly avoid rehospitalization. And finally, it may be useful for the patient to review his hospitalization by being able to identify (a) his maladaptive behaviors upon admission, (b) the environmental stresses that contributed to these symptoms, (c) what factors or experiences were responsible for his improvement, and (d) more effective ways he may respond to future stresses.

Another important yet obvious task of aftercare preparations is for the staff, in consultation with the patient and the significant people in his future environment, to determine the most appropriate *date of discharge*. In reaching this decision a number of factors need to be considered. Some of these include (a) the patient's behavior both in the hospital and on passes in the community, (b) the behavior of those in the patient's social network vis-à-vis the patient, (c) adequate aftercare planning, and (d) unfortunately, financial considerations. Hogarty (1972) has devised a Discharge Readiness Inventory which may assist clinicians in determining if a patient is actually ready to enter the community. In reaching a decision to discharge a patient the critical task is not setting a date, but rather determining if the patient is *ready* to leave the hospital by a specific date. By "ready" we mean to imply that the patient is able to live a productive and relatively self-satisfying existence within the community. Studies have shown that although many discharged patients are living in the community, this "community" is in many respects no different than the hospitals they came from (Lamb 1971). For example, the dreariness of a boarding home may not only have very few advantages over the boring routine of some hospitals, but may also have a number of disadvantages, such as lack of supervision, inadequate medical care, etc. Thus, the hospital staff must not only set a discharge date, but more importantly, they must try to determine if the patient is actually ready to leave the hospital and will be able to enter a supportive community environment.

Planning for Professional Outpatient Therapy

In many hospitals aftercare planning involves little more than finding a suitable outside therapist for the patient. We have purposely delayed a discussion of this activity until now, so that we may emphasize that aftercare preparation consists of a great deal more than simply choosing a therapist. The patient may see the doctor for one hour a week; he lives in the rest of the community for the remaining 167 hours. Therefore, the bulk of aftercare planning should attend to this latter consideration. Nevertheless, the referral to an outside therapist requires considerable fore-thought and careful implementation, if it is to be reactive to the patient's needs.

In making referral decisions the staff needs to consider (a) what type of treatment modality would be preferable, (b) who should conduct it, and (c) what is the priority of treatment issues. In reaching these deteminations several guidelines may be of assistance. Referral decisions should be made in consultation with the patient. It is important to know before rather than after the fact that Mrs. A detests Dr. B, or that Mrs. C dislikes group therapy. Whatever referral is made, it should begin, whenever possible, *before* the patient is discharged. This is especially true if the patient is starting with a new therapist. The patient may feel that her future doctor is unsympathetic, unreliable, or gen-erally offensive. If so, it is unlikely that the patient will continue to see that practitioner and may discontinue therapy soon after discharge. Therefore, while the patient is still in the hospital, he should have at least an initial trial visit with his outside therapist. Immediately following this interview, the hospital staff should carefully discuss with the patient what had transpired during the session in order to detect any possible difficulties that may have arisen. Similarly, the staff should talk to the outside therapist to obtain his assessment of the meeting, and then discuss with both the patient and the therapist what had occurred during this ini-tial session; potential problems may thus be avoided. Although ultimate effectiveness of formal outpatient therapy may, to a large extent, rest with the skills of the therapist, the hospital staff can do several things to ensure the likelihood of its success. In addi-tion to thoroughly discussing the patient's problems and treat-ment with the outside therapist, staff in making the referral can apprise the patient of a few important considerations. First, out-patient treatment is different from inpatient treatment and the therapist may not behave exactly like hospital personnel do. Sec-ond, unlike the inpatient staff the outside therapist may not be readily available on a 24-hour-a-day basis. Third, a new therapist is essentially a stranger to the patient, and a "get acquainted" period may be necessary before therapy can get into full gear. Of course, this latter problem may be obviated, if members of the hospital staff provide the follow-up treatment. Nevertheless, there are times when this is neither possible nor desirable. For example, in rural areas geographical factors may preclude the hospital staff from conducting outpatient treatment. In other instances the patient's resentment of or excessive dependency upon hospital personnel may serve as a contraindication for members of the staff to follow the patient after discharge.

Given our present state of knowledge, it is difficult to recommend to patients a particular follow-up treatment modality with any degree of certitude. Nevertheless, if the patient has participated in a variety of therapeutic procedures within the hospital, the staff can make a recommendation based upon its observations as to which treatment modality seemed most beneficial to the patient. Similarly, the patient, having been exposed to these numerous therapies, will have some firsthand knowledge as to what he feels has been most helpful. Of course, simply liking a treatment technique does not mean that it necessarily will be the most responsive to a patient's needs. For example, Sadoff (1971) has found that criminals who disliked group psychotherapy had a better long-term adjustment than those who preferred group therapy. In any event the decision as to which type of follow-up treatment a patient should have is a complex but important one, that needs careful planning and negotiation *before* discharge.

AFTERCARE PROGRAMS

Although the vast majority of hospitalized patients will be discharged to their homes and in the care of an outside therapist, others may benefit from other forms of rehabilitation. These may include Alcoholics Anonymous, drug treatment centers, Recovery Incorporated (a patient self-help group), other types of hospitalization, half-way houses, sheltered workshops, and so forth. Recently, with the increasing desire to maintain previously hospitalized individuals within the community a number of innovative aftercare programs have been devised.

Fairweather and his associates (1964, 1967) implemented a project whereby groups of chronically hospitalized patients would be gradually moved into a *community lodge*. Their patient sample consisted of long-term institutionalized patients who had lived together for a sufficient duration of time and had become mutually supportive to one another. They no longer possessed any family or friends with whom they could live. Their only associates were those individuals within the hospital milieu. Initially, in the hospital, and then eventually in the community lodge, the patients were expected to live together, work together, and play together. Each member of the group was trained while in the hospital to perform specific tasks that would eventually contribute to the overall maintenance of the lodge. Thus, some learned to prepare food, others to perform landscaping chores, and still others to clean the house. A system of rewards was developed wherein positive reinforcers were dispensed contingent upon each patient fulfilling his individual responsibility. It was also necessary for the patients to participate in income producing activities and to be trained to do so. The staff was also very careful in selecting the location of the community lodge, ensuring that the surrounding neighborhood would not be hostile to the program. Although the entire project is too complex to discuss here, the point is that groups of patients were prepared within the hospital to perform tasks necessary to live on the outside. In turn they were collectively transferred to a community lodge, where they participated in a living-working situation. Not only has this program continued to function successfully, but over 30 other community lodges have been established (Sanders 1973).

Another interesting project is the establishment of *Landlord-Supervised Cooperative Apartments* which are a hybrid of foster family care and independent apartment living. In these programs individual patients who are usually without a home are discharged to a community-based apartment that is supervised by a professionally trained landlord. The hospital provides back-up psychiatric and medical care in the form of home visits. The patients have expressed considerable satisfaction with these programs because they can enjoy its family atmosphere, yet maintain some privacy and independence. Another one of its major advantages is that, in comparison to other community-based facilities, such as half-way houses, the Landlord-Supervised Cooperative Apartments are highly economical (Chien 1973).

An imaginative program that can supplement other types of aftercare arrangements has been the *re-entry group*. Recently discharged patients meet for six to ten weekly sessions in a group conducted by patients previously released from the same unit. The ex-patient leaders, having evidenced a successful adjustment to community life, are trained in group procedures by members of the hospital staff. By having former inpatients leading the groups recently discharged individuals were able to see patients who had "made it" and were able to share their feelings of loneliness and futility with someone who had had similar experiences, and yet "survived" (Bachman 1971). Ex-patient leaders felt good about their participation not only because they were behaving as competent individuals, but also because the recently discharged patients would pay them for their services (Houpt 1972).

By way of review this chapter has presented some general guidelines for aftercare planning. It has suggested that aftercare planning become an integral part of the total hospital program, beginning on the day of admission and continuing throughout the remainder of hospitalization. The need for patients to exhibit behaviors that are both tolerated by and useful for society has been emphasized. The importance of teaching patients to be responsive to the typical reward and punishment patterns of their particular subculture has been noted. It has also been proposed that rehabilitation programs initiated within the hospital may be extended to the patient's home, if those with whom he lives are properly trained to carry it out. The need for a gradual transition from hospital to community, as well as several programs designed to accomplish this, has been discussed. And finally, several guidelines in arranging for follow-up treatment are suggested.

Although this chapter is the final one of part III, in a sense it is the most important. Unless aftercare procedures are thoroughly planned and carefully implemented, all of the fancy and imaginative hospital therapies will be of little ultimate value to the patient. It is easy to lose sight of this fact, since most staff only see the patient during the in-hospital phase of their rehabilitation. Nevertheless, the importance of effective aftercare planning cannot be overestimated. Unfortunately, there remains a great deal to be learned about how to carry out aftercare procedures, and, therefore, definitive conclusions as to how to implement such plans require further investigation.

Part IV

ADDITIONAL PREREQUISITES
OF A REACTIVE ENVIRONMENT

UP TO THIS POINT we have discussed the strictly clinical functions of a hospital staff. Nevertheless, several questions remain that need to be examined. How can the hospital staff be trained to provide high-quality clinical care? How will the staff know that its treatment techniques are achieving the desired results? How can the unit's record keeping system serve to enhance rather than to detract from the hospital's educational, research, and evaluative functions? Chapter 15 will attempt to answer these and other questions that are necessary, if a psychiatric hospital is to become a reactive environment.

Chapter 15

TRAINING, RESEARCH, EVALUATION, AND RECORD KEEPING

EVEN THOUGH we no longer chain and bleed our mentally ill, we may be subjecting them to a new and more subtle form of oppression—an oppression that arises from an unquestioning acceptance of our treatment methods. Despite the fact that many mental health workers tackle their work with zeal, they often preface their responses to questions of treatment effectiveness with statements such as, "I believe," or "that's just the way it's always done," etc. Combating ignorance disguised as benevolence is a difficult, but not an impossible, task. A climate of inquiry which is supported through continuous evaluation, research, and staff training is a formidable opponent of the mindless acceptance of the status quo. No contemporary psychiatric hospital staff can properly function if it is untrained and does not critically examine what it is doing both to and for patients.

Training, research, evaluation, and record keeping are brought together in this chapter because of their interdependence. In contradistinction to an untrained staff we feel that well-taught hospital personnel are better able to evaluate what they have done and are doing for patients. A trained staff, accustomed to evaluating their activities, are better prepared to ask and to research questions concerning the comparative effectiveness of different treatment variables. And finally, in order to evaluate one's treatment efforts and to conduct clinical research, a hospital staff must utilize an effective record keeping system.

TRAINING STAFF

Great confusion exists about training. We hear much about "new careers," "career ladders," but little about how they apply to the specific aspects of patient care. We believe that the training of those who work in a psychiatric unit should be directed towards aiding staff to perform its tasks more knowledgeably. Unfortunately, this is not always identical with acquiring high school equivalency certificates or college degrees. A relevant education is directed towards what staff actually do. In other words training must enhance not only the staff's patient care skills, but also its satisfaction in performing these tasks.

To maximize the likelihood of achieving both these goals, educational programs for hospital personnel should consider four related aspects. First, training courses ought to emphasize concrete practical skills consistent with what staff actually do on the unit; it differs from an exclusively theoretical discourse on patient care that seeks to primarily impart abstract knowledge. Second, the goals of the teaching experience should be clear to every participant. In this regard it is important to delineate the purposes of training. Third, attention must be paid to the methods employed in teaching. How can one teach what one feels is important? Fourth, and perhaps most neglected, it is necessary to consider possible ways of maintaining and reinforcing desirable staff behavior in relation to patients; this requires a constant attention to the continued application of the skills derived from training. We feel that each of these aspects is vital to any successful hospital staff teaching program.

In general the content of a training experience for staff should include the following: (a) familiarity with the language used for describing and discussing patients on the unit, (b) skill in observing interactions between patients, family members, and staff, (c) knowledge of how to behave with patients, especially those who are delusional, hallucinating, etc.; knowledge of how to intervene in various difficult situations, such as dealing with the agitated patient or one who refuses to take medication, (d) information concerning the predominant treatment modalities used on the unit, including both specific as well as theoretical data on the rationale for and the limitations of these methods, and (e) information about other programs in the hospital or available in nearby settings, e.g., geriatric care, drug abuse treatment, etc.

As already stated, what one desires to teach should be clearly delineated. For example, the general goal of teaching the staff of a behavior therapy unit might be to have them learn to design and to implement a specific behavior modification program for a particular patient. A clarification of this goal could result in the development of sub-goals, such as teaching staff to define specific target behaviors and to observe as well as to record their frequencies; to administer tokens contingent on desired activities of the patient; to monitor all changes in the patient's behavior; to determine the causal effectiveness of the treatment procedures (see below); to follow up on the breadth and the durability of change.

Once goals become clear so do the methods to attain them. Various approaches may be used for staff teaching. To continue with an example from the behaviorist camp, Gardner (1972) compared the efficacy of lecturing with what he termed "role playing" in terms of strengthening the behavior modification expertise of attendants working in an institution for the retarded. He found that lecturing was more successful in producing verbally sophisticated technicians, but role playing was more efficient in building better performance skills. A growing literature on paraprofessional and non-professional training in behavior modification suggests the value of combining methods, such as lecturing, providing assigned readings with study questions, demonstrating the correct practices, rehearsing these procedures, having discussion sessions, and giving homework assignments (Patterson 1970a, Poser 1972, LeBow 1973).

The fourth concern, the problem of the best way to *maintain* a high level of staff performance after a formal teaching program ends, involves the concept of staff reinforcement. The most effective way to maintain the occurrence of any behavior is to reward it. This principle and its relation to the continuation of important staff efforts has already been discussed in chapter 6.

Staff Sensitivity Training

In recent years the goal of high level patient care has been related to staff sensitivity training. Teaching hospital personnel to become more "sensitive" has become so prevalent in psychiatric units around the country that any contemporary treatise on hospital care should discuss this approach and attempt to place it into its proper perspective.

Utilizing encounter group techniques, sensitivity sessions are purported to enhance intra-staff communication and to cultivate self-awareness. Theoretically at least, it is expected that this activity will eventually pay off in terms of improved patient care.

The rationale for staff sensitivity groups is based upon observations made by clinicians of diverse theoretical orientations. Freud continuously stressed the need for psychoanalysts to examine their own unconscious motivation when dealing with patients. As a result, a personal analysis has been required for all therapists aspiring to become psychoanalysts. Nevertheless, it was the social psychiatrists who provided the major impetus for the establishment of sensitivity groups. By encouraging staff to assume a more egalitarian position vis-à-vis patients, Maxwell Jones (1953) has emphasized the need for hospital personnel to scrutinize their own feelings and behaviors within a clinical setting. Stanton and Schwartz (1954), T. F. Main (1957), and others have suggested that covert and unresolved intra-staff conflicts may result in compromised patient care. Discussions and resolution of these tensions were felt to be necessary in order to prevent these conflicts from eventually hindering patient treatment. Furthermore, the trend towards reducing traditional role dichotomies between patients and staff suggested that, if therapy is good for the patient, it also is good for the staff. Some therapists have conceptualized the unit's staff as being the patient's "alter-family" (Sager 1972a). Whitaker (1971) sees the total staff and patient sectors as representing a "tribe," with the staff being the parents and the patients being the children. As family therapists, both Sager and Whitaker reflexively prescribe family therapy, hence, staff sensitivity groups. With the increasing popularity of the "encounter culture," sensitivity training has been judged by many to be an indispensable experience for all those who work in organizational, and especially in hospital settings. And finally, the increasing importance ascribed to communications theory and group training has led to the incorporation of group experiences as part of professional psychiatric training programs (Redlich 1969).

A coalescence of these trends has given rise to a situation wherein staff sensitivity groups oftentimes are assumed to be a necessary experience for all hospital personnel. Unfortunately, this conviction frequently has led to situations in which staff become preoccupied with their own encounter groups and apparently forget that treatment is for the patients. For example, in reading Sager's account (1972a) of what he feels to be a successful staff sensitivity group one cannot help noticing that his staff is constantly engaged in tumultuous in-fighting. Sager's unlimited enthusiasm for his sensitivity groups leaves us with the impression that he prefers to focus upon conflict rather than work, staff self-awareness, rather than patient treatment. The assumption that sensitivity groups improve patient care has never been demonstrated. The effectiveness of T-group experience in managerial training and development would indicate that although the participants' behavior tends to change, job performance does not improve (Underwood 1965, Campbell 1968). We are not implying that staff sensitivity groups are without merit, but only that their goals need to be circumscribed and their use needs to be limited.

Although we do not share Abrom's (1971a) enthusiasm for staff sensitivity groups, we do appreciate his attempt to place their role within some kind of rational perspective. He suggests three general guidelines for their utilization. First, whatever is discussed should be clearly relevant to the staff's collaborative efforts in treating patients. The sessions are not to be a forum in which staff receive on-the-job psychotherapy. Second, only the leader of the group is permitted to render psychodynamic formulations. Other staff are to limit their comments to personal feelings and behavioral observations. This rule is intended to minimize the efforts of those group members more sophisticated in psychodynamics to use such dynamics as a "weapon" against other members. Third, the leader should not have any particular axe to grind regarding the unit's treatment program. He should not use his authority in order to favor one discipline or to influence the theoretical persuasion of the hospital's program (Abroms 1971a).

Although these guidelines may diminsh the possibility that staff sensitivity groups will become distracted from their ultimate mission (i.e., helping patients), they readily can be abused. Our concern over the inadequacy of his guidelines becomes heightened when in the same article Abroms states, "When staff members... are able to joke and reminisce together, only the *relatively small problem* of treating the patients remains." (Abroms 1971a, pp. 144-145) (authors' italics). While we are sure that Abroms does not literally believe that statement, we are concerned that many hospital staff behave as if they wholeheartedly embrace it.

Our *impression* is that oftentimes the demand by the staff for sensitivity groups arises when they become dissatisfied with their work. This disenchantment especially occurs when a unit's leadership fails to (a) provide the staff with adequate reinforcement for their therapeutic efforts, (b) offer ample opportunities to develop their professional skills, or (c) "take charge" in moments of crisis. In other words the need for sensitivity groups may emerge when leaders fail to lead. On the other hand when staff members are expanding their professional competencies, feel rewarded for their efforts, and trust their leaders, they enjoy their work and function as a cohesive and dedicated group.

Nevertheless, even under the best of circumstances the tensions of working with difficult patients (and difficult staff) can occasionally disrupt a normally unified staff. When this occurs, ad-hoc discussions of the existing conflicts may be invaluable in resolving intra-staff conflicts. Ad-hoc discussions, however, are a far cry from the permanent utilization of sensitivity groups, wherein staff contemplate and scrutinize each other's "vibrations" under the guise of being a legitimate training experience.

Our caution about sensitivity groups should not be extended to other group training methods. "Study groups" (Rice 1965, Astrachan 1969) may be of outstanding value in helping staff understand group phenomena and authority relationships. Those hospital personnel who will be conducting group therapy or psychodrama sessions may become more effective leaders, if they have had direct experiences in these types of groups. Even these types of experiential exercises, unfortunately, can become so emotionally draining that they can distract the staff's attention from patient care. If so, it is the responsibility of the unit's leadership to ensure that staff returns to its work, even if this means terminating the group experience.

Pierce and his collaborators (1972) have described a group method for expanding the staff's awareness of the hospital's program by utilizing the Ward Atmosphere Scale. This instrument measures ten dimensions of a unit's culture, such as clarity of communication, use of insight, degree of aggressiveness, etc. Each staff member is asked to rate these factors according to how he presently perceives the unit to be and how he feels ideally the unit should be. The discrepancy between these two ratings is discussed by the entire staff with the purpose of altering the present ward so it more closely approximates the ideal ward. Such a method may also help to define specific training objectives.

Well-trained personnel can maximize the successful operation of the hospital system. Conversely, poorly taught staff not only underutilize the therapeutic potential of the unit, but also make it detrimental to the welfare of the patient. That a hospital's personnel wittingly or unwittingly may have a deteriorative influence on patient functioning has been suggested by several researchers (Stanton 1954, Ayllon 1964, Gelfand 1967). Once staff more completely understands the mechanics of what it is doing with patients, it is in a better position to evaluate the success of these activities as well as to research relevant questions pertaining to its members. A very useful methodology, which is not only serviceable in orienting and training new staff but also advantageous in providing them with a consistent vocabulary, is standardized data collection.

RECORD KEEPING

It cannot be overemphasized that attention to the record keeping functions of a psychiatric service is important, because it provides a focus for both training and treatment. Grant and Maletzky (1972) have summarized the objectives of keeping psychiatric records as follows: (a) An adjunct to the staff's memory in terms of history, observations, as well as past and present treatment intervention. This also serves as a source of information sharing for the rest of the staff. (b) A readily accessible repository of up-to-date information. (c) A reflection of what actual treatment is taking place. (d) A record of the development and testing of clinical hypotheses. This function in itself is extremely important in creating a treatment and research climate on the unit. (e) A resource for elaborate clinical investigations. (f) A document available for scrutiny for both teaching and supervision purposes, as well as for medical audit. (g) An accurate legal document.

The surge of new interest in data processing and computer storage of information has helped in the development of new record keeping innovations. Two presently fashionable approaches are to collect data along the lines of a specific format, e.g., the problem-oriented record (Weed 1969), and to gather information with the aid of an interrelated series of forms, e.g., the Spitzer forms (Spitzer 1965, Endicott 1972), the KDS system (Kupfer 1971b), or the ECDEU assessment manual (Guy 1970).

Problem-Oriented Record

The problem-oriented record (Weed 1969, Grant 1972) consists of four major components: the data base, the problem list, the initial plan, and the progress note. The *data base*, which ordinarily is present in the admission note, may include any or all of the following: chief complaint, patient profile and related social data, present and past psychiatric and medical history, results from physical and mental status examinations, and preliminary reports of laboratory and psychological tests. Information garnered from the patient, as well as from significant others in his social matrix, should be included within the data base. In writing this as well as all other portions of the record it is important to categorize separately *subjective data* (i.e., what the patient or his family says) and *objective data*, (i.e., what the staff observes or the laboratory reports).

The *problem list* functions as the central skeleton upon which all subsequent entries are based. It consists of all the patient's psychiatric and medical problems, whether past or present. As Weed states, "the list should not contain diagnostic guesses; it should simply state the problems at a level of refinement consistent with the physician's understanding, running the gamut from the precise diagnosis to the isolated, unexplained finding." (Weed 1969, p. 25) The problem list is derived from the information included in the data base. An example of a problem list is seen in Table VIII. As hospitalization proceeds, new problems, as well as the dates on which they occur, may be added to the list (see Table VIII, #7), while other problems can be changed to an inactive status.

TABLE VIII
Sample Problem List (6/5/73)

ACTIVE PROBLEMS

1. Depression
   a. crying spells
   b. psychomotor retardation
   c. expression of self-denigrating statements
2. Marital conflict
   a. frequent verbal feuds
   b. threatened divorce
3. Poor eye contact
4. Right upper quadrant mass, questionable

7. Loss of job (6/17/73)

INACTIVE PROBLEMS

5. Elevator phobia
6. Barbiturate abuse

TABLE IX
Sample Initial Plan

1. *Depression*
   imipramine, 150 mg. at h.s.
   encourage activity
   positive expression of self-esteem
   obtain more detailed history of patient's development
2. *Marital conflict*
   family assessment
3. *Poor eye contact*
   encourage direct eye contact by means of positive reinforcement
4. *Right upper quadrant mass, questionable*
   urinalysis
   flat plate and upright
   intravenous pyelogram

The *initial plans* should be numbered according to the specific category on the problem list. Table IX illustrates an initial plan based on the problems enumerated on Table VIII. As can be seen, the plans may include either further assessment or treatment interventions.

The *progress notes* consist of recordings of a follow-up of each of the problems delineated in the problem list. They are subdivided according to subjective data, objective data, assessment data (i.e. a discussion of the problem), and additional plans.

Although a more detailed discussion of the problem-oriented record can be found elsewhere (Weed 1969, Grant 1972), several of its virtues are worth mentioning. In systematically reviewing each of the problems and the plans for resolving them by means of regular progress notes, very little can be overlooked, at least regarding initial impressions. The problem-oriented record is a clear, almost stepwise, progression in the care of the patient. Consequently, in most hospitals at which it has been instituted, after an initial period of unfamiliarity and thereby resistance to it (Lipsius 1973), most people feel that it is an extremely efficient method for systematizing patient care, assessing treatment, and training staff. Another advantage of this system is that it can operate primarily on the basis of behavior manifested by the patient, even to the exclusion of diagnostic categories. At times diagnostic categories tend to restrict thinking about the patient's condition and create a type of "tunnel vision," whereas the problem-oriented record allows one to make precise behavioral observations of the patient. Although the problem-oriented system has been more widely used in medical and surgical care, it is being increasingly adapted for psychiatric services.

The utility of the problem-oriented record for psychiatric hospital personnel could be enhanced even further if it were to have a more explicit way of incorporating treatment objectives into the system. One could speak of a "goal-oriented record," wherein the problems are designated as in Table VIII, but in addition a set of goals for hospitalization in the rehabilitation of each one of these problems is specifically determined. For example, the goal for crying spells (Problem #1a) may be the total absence of such behavior, while for marital conflicts (Problem #2) the inpatient goal may be only to assess the situation and to arrange for long-term outpatient couples therapy. The advantage of adding a goal-oriented approach is that it may help the inpatient staff to clearly specify its treatment objectives. All too often hospital personnel become disillusioned because the patient does not leave the unit as "a paragon of mental health," having retained significant behavior problems. In these circumstances it is useful for the staff to be able to distinguish between the objectives of in and outpatient care. The systematic designation of goals as part of the problem-oriented record might assist in achieving this purpose.

Standardized Inter-Connected Data Collection Systems

Perhaps the most widely known data collection approach in psychiatry is the one devised by Spitzer and his collaborators (e.g. 1965, 1970, Endicott 1972). This system includes a psychiatric anamnestic record, various daily ratings, and symptom status forms. All of these instruments are available for computerized scoring and can give printouts on all the information collected, as well as the diagnostic categories that such data suggests. This system also has training films and manuals which provide for the development of high degrees of inter-rater reliability. Additionally, several other systems have been devised (Lorr 1962, Overall 1962, Guy 1970, Kupfer 1971b). Although these systems are of use in a general way, when there are specific research interests or particular problems of a hospital, many of these forms have to be modified. These forms, at least those for data collection, can complement the problem-oriented record and provide a standardized data base for both information retrieval and clinical research. Because these forms possess a high inter-rater reliability, they also can be used for inter-hospital drug efficacy studies. Furthermore, they can provide a convenient training vehicle by increasing the staff's observational skills. This can be achieved by reviewing and comparing each staff member's ratings in a group setting.

From the above description of these types of record and data collection systems, their clinical utility and potential for creating an atmosphere of inquiry becomes immediately apparent. First, by recording data in this manner forgotten or neglected information may be discovered. Second, when one uses such data collection systems, the patient's more prominent symptoms are immediately highlighted. This enables the staff to identify and to focus upon the patient's behavior problems. Third, such standardization allows the staff to compare and to classify patients. Fourth, if the same rating scales are used as part of follow-up procedures, there is a baseline provided to measure change. Fifth, one can use these scales to measure patients' behavior and compare treatment interventions. Sixth, they are extremely useful in terms of training and orienting new staff, as well as for providing a consistent vocabulary for the existing staff. Seventh, the use of such rating systems, if they are attended to by the unit directors, may help to create for the staff a climate of inquiry and feedback. In other words, without adding unnecessarily to the staff's workload, the use of these instruments may considerably enhance the clinical, educational, and investigatory functions of the psychiatric hospital.

RESEARCH AND EVALUATION

Unfortunately, for some the terms "research" and "evaluation" conjure up images of elaborate experimentation and expensive laboratory equipment. In their most basic sense, however, research and evaluation mean studious inquiry, diligent searching, and careful examination. This view of research and evaluation can be of major importance to the care of patients. Clinicians, not just academicians, must see research and evaluation within their scope of patient centered activities. Essentially, we are saying that a psychiatric unit should create and maintain an atmosphere of critical examination, research, and inquiry.

A common belief among many mental health professionals is that research and good clinical care are incompatible. In its most bland form this view is manifested when clinicians object to research and evaluation on the grounds that they do not have time for these activities. In our view clinicians do not have time to avoid them. A more strenuous objection, though not often voiced, results perhaps from the fear of examining one's clinical efforts or scrutinizing the value of one's education, an education that has taken years to acquire. Often the preconceptions of the mentor are passed from one generation to another, and become solidly entrenched in clinical practice so that the clinician never examines his basic conceptions. The results are, in any case, the same. Upon examination, one often finds that frequently practiced techniques show little evidence to justify their continued use. In a progressive psychiatric unit which questions and examines its methods patient care will ultimately improve.

Both evaluation and research in the psychiatric hospital seek to answer questions about treatment variables. Whereas evaluation attempts to find out whether treatment techniques used by staff are effective for the particular patients receiving them, research attempts to formulate and to answer new questions about the worthiness of various treatment variables *per se*. Answering evaluation and research questions requires some knowledge of experimental design. Group and single-subject design represent two types of methodology serviceable to hospital personnel for most questions of evaluation and research.

Group design research usually results from a decision to study a specific aspect of the rehabilitation program, a particular type of patient problem, or differing roles of staff. In these cases one defines how many subjects are needed (groups) and how this population will be studied. For example, if one wants to investigate the efficacy of treatment A versus treatment B, one would need to have a different group of patients who received each treatment. In addition one might want to control for the effect of no treatment at all and would select a group (C) who received neither approach. Other controls are possible. The differing treatments (A and B) and no treatment are independent variables—that is, they are the quantities that are varied. To assess the effects of these independent variables, one needs some measure, such as patient behavior, as to what are the effects of treatment A versus treatment B versus no treatment on the same behavior of each group of patients? Behavior then becomes the dependent variable. Patients assigned to each group must be similar in terms of the behavior (s) dealt with and have no major differences (e.g., intelligence or sex) that could bias the results and make them difficult to interpret.[1] After data from the experiment is gathered, it is usually subjected to statistical manipulations so that conclusions may then be drawn.

Group design research and evaluation present problems in a clinical setting. It is difficult, for instance, to find large enough groups of subjects similar in critical ways before treatment; this requirement must be fulfilled in order to minimize interpretive problems. But group comparisons can be carried out. In some psychiatric units, where a strong research interest exists, investigation can be formalized. In these situations research may be looked upon as an aspect of the treatment program in which data is used not only to evaluate the treatment but also to illuminate other aspects of the patient's behavior. For example, some units as Tompkins-I (see chapter 5) have a regular time slot, such as one morning a week, set aside for the patients to fill out a series of forms which reflect certain specific changes in their behaviors. Within this framework of investigation various groups of patients can be formed *and then be studied for specific symptoms or responses to treatment.* The works of May (1964) and Shanfield (1970) exemplify this mode of investigation with patients diagnosed as schizophrenic. Although perhaps these research formats are more elaborate than most units require, they are well suited to and can be instituted for a specific project. On an ongoing basis, however, such an approach requires a nearly full-time staff member who can coordinate the operation (e.g., which patients receive which tests at which time, who will score the tests, what tests no longer serve a useful purpose, etc.).

A methodology that does not require large groups of subjects for research and evaluation purposes, and one that can fit into the ongoing activities of all staff design, is the single-subject. Behavior therapists have been most responsible for its extension and refinement in a clinical setting.

Single-subject designs can help to answer several questions, the

---

[1] The group design necessitates that individuals are randomly assigned to treatment groups (see Winer 1962) .

most salient one being, "Do the techniques I use work?" This query is not answered by simply observing that patients get better, for they may change for reasons unrelated to the treatment they receive. Evaluating whether a particular treatment is responsible for a particular positive alteration in the patient's behavior can be accomplished in several ways.

The two approaches presented below are particularly well suited to the clinician's activities. These methods may be employed for evaluating the treatment given to one or several patients who are not randomly assigned to different treatment conditions, as is typically done in an experiment using a group design. Suppose, for example, that one desires to increase the number of times a patient talks with his peers. It is observed that the patient seems to be responsive to praise from the staff. Therefore, it is decided that each time the patient is found conversing with other patients, a staff member will praise him (e.g., "It seems like you are having a nice conversation, Mr. G, I like what you are doing," etc.).

The reversal design. To evaluate the effectiveness of praise as a treatment variable, staff must impose several conditions. The major purpose of all these conditions is to show that because the treatment procedure is operative, a change in behavior occurs in the sought after direction. More specifically, in our example, when the patient is praised for talking with peers, the number of times he engages in this behavior increases. To say that behavior increases or decreases requires that one establish a reference point—in this case a pre-treatment period of observation (see chapter 6) during which the number of times the patient is found to be talking with his peers is tabulated. This is the first condition of the reversal method. During this *baseline* phase observers try to register the frequency of talking without attempting to influence it unduly.[1]

After baseline data is gathered, the *treatment condition is pre-*

---

[1] Observing behavior, however, undoubtedly affects it (see S. M. Johnson 1973).

sented. Thus, each time the patient is seen conversing, he is praised. Observations of the frequency of this behavior are continued for awhile, and one finds that the patient begins to talk more often to other patients. It is reasonable to ask, however, whether praise or some other variable (a chance variable) is responsible for the positive alteration in the behavior. To lend any credence to the assertion that giving praise is responsible for the desired behavior change, one must *temporarily discontinue* it and then observe whether conversing decreases in frequency. Thus, the third condition, in effect, reinstates the baseline phase for short periods of time in order to see if the behavior returns to its pre-treatment level. After the alteration occurs, the *treatment procedure should be applied once again* so that the desirable behavior will be recovered. By employing these four conditions, therefore, one can evaluate whether the treatment variable is effective in causing change in the patient's behavior. Variants of this reversal method of evaluation exist (see Sherman 1969).

Several problems with the reversal method prevail (Bandura 1969, Kazdin 1972b). Two major ones are that the particular target behaviors may not reverse after they have been altered, and that the staff may not reinstate treatment, even temporarily. With regard to the former handicap it is certainly possible, even desirable, for a behavior, once altered positively, to remain that way. If a patient is praised for conversing with his peers and these conversations become rewarding in and of themselves, as well as instrumental to the patient's obtaining other reinforcers (e.g., he learns how to do things), it is unlikely that removing the staff's praise will result in a decrement in the patient's conversations. In this particular situation praise from the staff may become unnecessary (see chapter 6). Clearly, the reversal method is inappropriate for evaluating the effectiveness of treatment when the target behavior does not reverse. Although this problem precludes the use of this method, objections to instituting reversals *per se* may be dealt with by stressing the importance of evaluation. Staff must be reassured that the reversal will only be temporary. Another way to deal with objections to the reversal method is to utilize, whenever possible, the following approach.

The multiple baseline design. This method (Baer 1968) also can be used to show that the treatment procedure is functional in changing the target behavior. This demonstration can be carried out if the treatment variable is applied at different points in time to several behaviors. Variations of this method can be found where, instead of different behaviors, different individuals are focused on, or the same person in different situations is dealt with (see Hall 1970b). With a multiple baseline method applied to one individual's various behaviors, one gathers several baselines concurrently—one for each behavior. Suppose that not only the frequency of conversing with other patients, but also the frequency of smiling at other patients except when he is conversing—two apparently independent behaviors—are tabulated. The treatment variable, e.g., praise, is then applied to one of these targets, e.g., speaking with patients. Once an increase in the frequency of this positive activity shows up, it is compared to the unchanged frequency of smiling, the second behavior. In short the altered behavior—talking with other patients—should be contrasted with the unaltered one—smiling except when in a conversation. A change in the frequency of talking in comparison to no marked change in the frequency of smiling should be evident. Then, the treatment variable is applied to the second target behavior and its change recorded; after this, other activities can be modified, and so forth. The effectiveness of the treatment variable is continually demonstrated by the changes which result in the target behaviors, when treatment is applied to each of them. By sequentially increasing the strength of talking and then doing the same to smiling, one gains confidence that praise is an effective treatment measure. This trust grows as other behaviors also are modified in the same manner. Therefore, with a multiple baseline design, several activities may be initially defined, observed, recorded, and subsequently, modified.

It is quite possible that the target behaviors selected for alterations are not independent. Thus, as one behavior is changed, the other behavior also is changed. For example, if one praises talking with peers and finds that it becomes stronger, one also might discover that the same change occurs with smiling at friends, even though this latter activity was not attended to specifically. When this circumstance takes place, one knows that the behaviors are not independent, and hence the multiple baseline is not appropriate by itself to evaluate the effectiveness of treatment. It is advisable in this case to employ, perhaps, a parametric analysis by which different amounts of praise are applied to see if the target behavior is differentially affected (Baer 1968). Or, a procedure in which different forms of the behavior are rewarded could be instituted (see LeBow 1973).

Evaluating the utility of treatment is not enough. It is also necessary to examine the durability of change; that is, one must eventually ascertain if the results which arise from treatment endure (see chapters 6 and 8).

It is clear that many of these formal designs require planning and concerted staff and patient effort in order to implement them successfully. Certainly, there may be segments of the staff that possess neither the time nor the inclination to be directly involved in these research endeavors. Nevertheless, it is valuable for those primarily engaged in such investigations to share information about their research with the remainder of the staff in order to stimulate a spirit of inquiry and curiosity. By so doing an atmosphere of clear and rational thinking may prevail, which ultimately will enhance the clinical care afforded psychiatric patients.

Appendix A

CONSTITUTION OF THE PATIENT ADVISORY BOARD

TOMPKINS-I (T-I) is a community comprised of all the patients and staff—a community whose credo is that people can learn to be responsible for themselves, and are able to help themselves through helping others.

I. *Purpose:*

The goal of the patient community of Tompkins-I is to encourage mutual responsibility among patients in exercising judgments for individual and group functioning, for the purpose of understanding themselves and others. The patient Advisory Board serves as a means of communication among patients and between the patient community and the staff.

II. *Patient Advisory Board:*

A. Membership:
1. The board is composed of nine patients who manifest responsible behavior; they are all elected by members of the patient community.

This constitution was written by the patients of Tompkins-I.

2. Election:
   a. One member is elected from each psychiatric resident's group every two weeks at a specified advisory board meeting.
   b. The remaining members are elected at large from the patient community.
   c. The chairman and vice-chairman of the advisory board are elected by and from the nine newly elected board members.
      1. When neither the chairman nor the vice-chairman is present, they may appoint replacements for themselves from the board. If this has not been done, the monitor for the day becomes the chairman pro-tempore and takes on their responsibilities.
   d. The secretary is a community member who volunteers for the position on those alternate weeks not devoted to the election of new board members.
   e. Procedure for the impeachment of chairman, vice-chairman, secretary, or member of the board may be started through a written request or a motion submitted verbally by a community member. The decision is made by community vote after sufficient discussion.
3. Term of Office:
   a. Two week office for board members and the secretary.
   b. There is no limit to the number of terms a chairman, vice-chairman, secretary, or member can serve.

B. Responsibilities:

1. Chairman
   a. To conduct meetings of the patient advisory board.

    b. To maintain order and to encourage participation in the meetings.

    c. To promote and to summarize discussion in the meetings.

    d. To vote when necessary to break a tie.

    e. To call emergency meetings when necessary.

    f. To make sure that up-to-date rules are posted and announcements are made.

2. Vice-Chairman

    a. To assist or to replace the chairman when necessary.

    b. To read and lead discussion on the chairman's pass request.

    c. To assign a sponsor (preferably from the Monitor Pool) to each new patient as soon as the monitor has notified him of a new patient's arrival.

3. Secretary

    a. The secretary is not a voting board member and may not resign as secretary to accept nomination to be a voting member of the board until his term of office expires.

    b. To write detailed minutes of all patient advisory board meetings.

    c. To present and to interpret the minutes when requested at patient-staff meetings.

    d. To prepare for the staff a mimeographed summary of requests, votes, and discussion items prior to patient-staff meetings.

    e. To give all minutes and pass requests to the recreational therapist who then files them.

4. Members of the Advisory Board

    a. To discuss and to vote responsibly and objectively on every issue with no members abstaining. If a member or members remain undecided, more discussion will take place to help them in their decision. If there remains any reasonable doubt in a member's mind after adequate discussion, he should vote negatively on a pass request.

b. To represent the viewpoints of other patients.

c. To make motions on discussion items and on status changes.

C. Procedures:

1. Meetings

a. Meetings will be held regularly at least three times a week.

b. An additional Friday meeting is held in order to set up for specials, checks, and monitors for the weekend. Status review is held for all patients up to Independent Status. Aside from this, no new passes may be submitted.

c. When necessary, the chairman may call an emergency meeting at any other time. The emergency nature of any passes submitted at such a meeting must be voted upon by the board.

d. The chairman must call a special meeting, if necessary, to consider the passes of those people unable to attend the regular meetings of the advisory board.

2. Attendance

a. Board members and all members of the patient community are required to attend unless someone is excused by the chairman for legitimate reasons, such as:

1. appointment with a doctor

2. outside therapy, work, or pleasure passes

3. an illness recognized by the staff

4. other special situations.

b. A quorum of seven voting members (six members and the vice-chairman) must be present in order to hold a meeting.

3. Passes

    a. Only patients on the Buddy System may apply for a pass, though in very special cases patients who are not on the Buddy System may be granted administrative passes by their doctor. A patient must be present at the meeting in which his pass or passes are discussed.

    b. Types of passes
        1. pleasure passes
            a. hourly, usually for dinner
            b. one day
            c. overnight
            d. weekend or double overnight
        2. work passes
        3. school passes
        4. outside therapy passes
        5. study passes.

    c. Mimeographed pass request forms are found in an envelope posted on the activities bulletin board. If there are no forms left, pass requests may be written on blank sheets of paper, as long as the format of the mimeographed pass requests is followed.

    d. Pass requests must accurately specify the times, days, and dates of a pass. Failure to do so may be cause for the chairman to rule the pass request out of order. A patient announces the purpose of his pass verbally at the advisory board meeting at which the request is taken up, and a pass may not be used for any other purpose than that specified.

    e. Pass requests must be deposited in the box on the counter at the nurses' station.

    f. Once the box is opened at a regular meeting, further requests may not be submitted. No requests may be submitted during meetings. Exceptions may be considered at the discretion of the chairman and the staff.

g. All pass requests (both those granted and those denied) are reviewed by the community at the next regularly scheduled patient-staff meeting. A pass that must be taken up before either of the two patient-staff meetings are convened, must be submitted to the board as an emergency pass request. An emergency pass request is reviewed and granted or rejected by signature of the patient's doctor.

h. No more than three passes may be submitted for review at a single patient-staff meeting. Exceptional cases will be considered at the discretion of the chairman of the advisory board and/or the staff.

i. No joint passes of community members may be submitted. Patients who wish to go out on a pass together must submit identical but separate passes, each of which will be considered on its individual merits or lack thereof.

4. Functions

a. The board regularly decides upon matters listed below but it is always flexible and open to new considerations. All board decisions are presented to the staff at patient-staff meetings and are subject to review by the staff at that time. Decisions made at the patient-staff meetings are final.

b. Patient status

1. patients may apply to the advisory board to be put on or taken off Staff Special, Patient Special, Ten-Minute Checks, Independent Status, the Monitor Pool and the Buddy System. These changes are made at the discretion of the board, and all changes are subject to approval by the staff.

2. patient status will be reviewed at all advisory board meetings, and changes may be made at the initiation of a board member, or of a member of the community.

c. The board will vote on all pass requests, and a majority vote of the board members is necessary for a pass request to be granted and presented for review at the patient-staff meeting.

d. Suggestions or recommendations concerning any ward problems, activities, or privileges are to be considered at board meetings.

e. Reconsideration of granted passes in light of new information or abuse of privileges will be at the discretion of the chairman or the staff.

f. Appointments of the daily monitors, checkers, and specialers for the following day or weekend shall be set up at regular advisory board meetings.

g. If there are more Monitor Pool assignments than there are patients on the Monitor Pool to fill them, the board may vote to place a patient onto "temporary Monitor Pool" to be able to special or check (not monitor). A patient is on temporary Monitor Pool for only as long as he is needed to fill Monitor Pool assignments.

h. The advisory board will attempt to abide by parliamentary procedure as much as possible.

i. Infractions involve irregularities of functioning on either the Monitor Pool or Buddy System.

1. Monitor Pool infractions: If it is felt that an infraction has been committed in any of the Monitor Pool responsibilities (specialing, checking, or monitoring), the problem will be discussed by a group consisting of a nurse, monitor, chairman, and the secretary of the board and the patient involved. After reviewing the issues they may

take immediate action (e.g. status change) if they consider this necessary. The advisory board will be informed of the decision at their next meeting and the decision will be listed on the patient-staff sheet. The patient is automatically grounded for 24 hours after a second infraction appears on the same patient-staff sheet.

2. Buddy System infractions: If it is felt that the infraction has been committed with respect to the Buddy System or on a pass, the problem will be discussed by a group consisting of the same people as above. After reviewing the issues, they may take immediate action (e.g. grounded from pass, grounded from walks, or status change). The advisory board will be informed of the decision and take any further action if necessary. The infraction will be listed on the patient-staff sheet. The patient is automatically grounded for 24 hours after a second infraction appears on the same patient-staff sheet.

3. Other irregularities: Irregularities on the ward will be dealt with in the same fashion as the above procedures for infractions. The problem will be discussed by the same group as above. Examples:
    1. Not signing in or out properly on the sheets
    2. Forgetting medications
    3. Returning late from pass

BY-LAWS *(abridged)*
MONITOR POOL

Patients must be on Independent Status in order to submit a pass request to the advisory board to be on the Monitor Pool. If the request is granted, they are then permitted to volunteer to be monitor, ten-minute checker, or patient specialer.

The chairman will have a list of those in the Monitor Pool at every advisory board meeting in order to set up specials, checkers, and monitors for the following day or weekend. Any failure to fulfill the responsibility of monitor, ten-minute checker, or patient specialer will result in review and action by the board. The chairman has the power to remove or replace any monitor, checker, or specialer. In the absence of the chairman, the vicechairman has the above power.

Whenever a monitor, checker, or specialer must leave his duties for other important activities, he must appoint a temporary substitute for himself from the Monitor Pool and inform the charge nurse and the monitor. This substitute must meet the same requirements (i.e., that of being on the monitor pool) and fulfill the same duties as the person for whom he substitutes. Under no circumstances may a patient serving as monitor, specialer, or checker use the Buddy System privileges at that time.

From time to time there will be Monitor Pool review to evaluate members of the Monitor Pool and to determine how they are functioning. The *monitor* is expected:

1. To attend reports at the nurses' station at 7:30 a.m. and at 3:30 p.m. Attendance at the 11:30 p.m. report is optional.
2. To awaken all patients at 7:15 a.m.
3. To assist the nurse in getting patients to blood pressures, temperatures, blood work, and medications.
4. To make sure that all patients attend meals, meetings, and activities on time unless they have a suitable excuse.

5. To play the role of host or hostess, doing everything possible to make guests feel at home during visiting hours and to ask guests to leave when visiting hours are over.

6. To enforce rules.

7. To be responsible for the general physical appearance of the ward.

8. To be aware of what is happening on the entire ward, and to share with the nurses any information about special problems or inappropriate behavior that may arise, and to give or to obtain assistance for patients in need of help.

9. To know which patients are on checks and specials and who their respective checkers and specialers are, and to inform the checker and specialers of important information brought up at nurses' report concerning their charges.

10. To inform the vice-chairman when a new patient is admitted in order to arrange for a sponsor as soon as possible after the new patient's arrival.

11. To assist in organizing and taking the patients to gym.

12. To organize and supervise patient attendance at chief's rounds.

13. To keep notes on Saturdays and Sundays and to prepare brief written notes on each patient, to be presented at the Monday morning patient-staff meeting.

14. All Monitor Pool duties are over at 10:00 p.m. at which time the staff assumes the ward responsibilities.

Ten-minute Checkers are expected:

1. To attend the 7:30 a.m. report at the nurses' station fully dressed for the day. Attendance at the 3:30 p.m. and 11:30 p.m. reports is optional.

2. To check every ten minutes on the whereabouts, and behavior of the patients assigned to them.

3. To refer any problems that may arise to the monitor or charge nurse.

4. To assist in taking the patients to gym.

When more than three patients are on checks, two checkers should be assigned.

The *patient specialer* is expected to stay with the patient assigned to him at all times except under the following circumstances.

- a. When the patient being specialed has a visitor, the specialer may leave him with the visitor with the understanding that the visitor is to return the patient to his specialer before leaving the floor.
- b. When the patient being specialed has an appointment with a staff member, said member should be informed that the patient is being specialed and is asked to return the patient to his specialer at the end of the meeting.

BUDDY SYSTEM

The regular Buddy System is an arrangement by which two or more patients may spend time off the ward by accepting responsibility for themselves and each other. Patients will be placed on Buddy System when they submit written passes to the advisory board which are approved by the board and by the staff in patient-staff meetings. Before applying for the Buddy System a patient must be on the Monitor Pool and must demonstrate responsibility as a monitor, checker, and patient specialer.

Rules of the Buddy System

1. Any patient who is on the Buddy System may leave the hospital with another patient of similar status unless a modification is imposed by the staff or the advisory board. Buddies may be away from the ward from after breakfast until 9:30 p.m. for no longer than three hours at a time. After 6:00 p.m. a buddy must be accompanied by two other buddies. Buddies may not miss meals, meetings, activities, medications, or blood pressures.

2. Buddies are expected to remain together at all times when out of the hospital. If for any reason this is not possible, the charge nurse should be informed at once.

3. Patients using the Buddy System privileges may not take any form of transportation unless they have permission from their doctor. If buddies find it necessary to take any form of transportation, they should notify the ward by telephone immediately.

Appendix B

GROUP THERAPY INFORMATION

People often feel uncomfortable their first time in group and don't know what is expected of them. This sheet is intended to give new members an introduction to what they should do in group therapy.

Group therapy is an important therapy for many people with emotional problems. It is prescribed for some and not for others, just as medications may or may not be prescribed. Groups are of different sizes and may include patients with varying ages and problems.

The task of the group is to help members learn more helpful ways to deal with their problems and feelings. People tend to use the same ways of dealing with other people in group that they use in their private lives. For instance, if the way someone behaves in the group makes you feel uncomfortable, it probably makes people in his private life also feel uncomfortable.

For example, Jack, a business man, looked angrily at any

This group information sheet (Rogoff 1973) was written for and is distributed to all patients at the Dartmouth-Hitchcock Mental Health Center (see chapter 4).

group member who did not agree with him. He used the same method outside the group with his wife and boss.

Also, a person who has difficulty speaking up in the group probably has difficulty speaking up in his private life.

For instance, JoAnn had difficulty talking with members of the group. At home she also had difficulty talking. Her friends felt uncomfortable about this and stopped visiting her. As a result, JoAnn was increasingly alone, which made her problems worse.

In both cases the person was unaware of the effect he had on others and how his behavior affected them. These people were helped when other people in the group told them how they were behaving.

Members also help each other by asking questions to find out more about each other, pointing out to others how they look or seem and sharing their own emotional reactions. Because you have problems does not mean that you can't help others.

Members don't help each other when they:

1) avoid tense subjects or change the issue when people become uncomfortable. Often it is necessary to talk about painful issues, if one wants to get better;

2) argue without trying to see what the other person is saying;

3) depend on the staff to tell them what to do;

4) talk to just one or a few of the patients in a group, shutting off the rest of the group;

5) talk about events that occurred outside the group and therefore can't be dealt with by the group.

For example, the group was talking about loneliness and Mary began to cry. They continued their discussion and ignored Mary. This was an unfortunate way to deal with the problem. Mary felt frustrated because she wanted to tell the group of her loneliness since the death of her mother. The group lost a chance to offer her support and advice on how to cope with her grief.

Another illustration was Bill who liked to talk about his childhood and rambled on for a long time about this during group. This was not helpful to Bill or to the other members of the group; and in doing so Bill lost a valuable opportunity to talk about his alcoholism which was the reason for his admission.

Therapists are there to help keep the group focused on the task.

Groups are frequently observed by other members of the staff involved in patient care and these observers give the therapists information and advice on how they have conducted their job. You will be notified if your doctor feels group therapy will be beneficial for you.

BIBLIOGRAPHY

ABROMS, G. M. (1968). Setting limits. *Archives of General Psychiatry,* 19:113-119.

ABROMS, G. M. (1969a). Defining milieu therapy. *Archives of General Psychiatry,* 21:553-560.

ABROMS, G. M. (1969b). Setting limits and teaching skills. In *Current Psychiatric Therapies,* ed. J. Masserman, New York: Grune and Stratton, 9:63-72.

ABROMS, G. M. (1971a). Group methods in the milieu. In *The New Hospital Psychiatry,* eds. G. M. Abroms and N. S. Greenfield, New York: Academic.

ABROMS, G. M., FELLNER, C. H., and WHITAKER, C. A. (1971b). The family enters the hospital. *Archives of General Psychiatry,* 127:1363-1370.

ACKERMAN, N. W. (1958). The Psychodynamics of Family Life. New York: Basic Books.

Action for Mental Health (1961). Final Report to the Joint Committee on Mental Illness and Health. New York: Basic Books.

AGRAS, W. S. (ed.) (1972a). Behavior Modification: Principles and Clinical Applications. Boston: Little, Brown, and Co.

AGRAS, W. S. (1972b). The behavioral therapies: underlying principles and procedures. In *Behavior Modification: Principles and Clinical Applications,* ed. W. S. Agras, Boston: Little, Brown, and Co.

AITCHISON, R. A. (1972). A low cost rapid delivery point system with 'automatic recording'. *Journal of Applied Behavior Analysis,* 5:527-528.

ALEXANDER, F. G., and SELESNICK, S. T. (1966). The History of Psychiatry: An Evaluation of Psychiatric Thought and Practice from Prehistoric Times to the Present. New York: Harper and Row.

ALMOND, R., KENISTON, K., and BOLTAX, S. (1968). The value system of a milieu therapy unit. *Archives of General Psychiatry,* 19:545-561.

261

ALMOND, R., KENISTON, K., and BOLTAX, S. (1969). Patient value change in milieu therapy. *Archives of General Psychiatry*, 20:339-351.

ALMOND, R. (1971). The therapeutic community. *Scientific American*, 224 (March): 34-42.

ASTRACHAN, B. M., HARROW, M., BECKER, R. E., SCHWARTZ, A. H., and MILLER, J. C. (1967). The unled patient group as a therapeutic tool. *International Journal of Group Psychotherapy*, 17:178-191.

ASTRACHAN, B. M., and REDLICH, F. C. (1969). Leadership ambiguity and its effect on resident's study groups. *International Journal of Group Psychotherapy*, 19:487-494.

ATTHOWE, J., and KRASNER, L. (1968). Preliminary report on the application of contingent reinforcement procedures (token economy) on a 'chronic' psychiatric ward. *Journal of Abnormal Psychology*, 73:-37-43.

AYD, F. (1966). Drug holidays—intermittent pharmacotherapy for psychiatric patients. *International Drug News Letter*, 1:8.

AYD, F. J. (1970). Prevention of recurrence (maintenance therapy). In *Clinical Handbook of Psychopharmacology*, eds. A. DiMascio and R. I. Shader, New York: Science House.

AYLLON, T., and MICHAEL, J. (1959). The psychiatric nurse as a behavioral engineer. *Journal of the Experimental Analysis of Behavior*, 2:323-334.

AYLLON, T. (1963). Intensive treatment of psychotic behavior by stimulous satiation and food reinforcement. *Behavior Research and Therapy*, 1:53-61.

AYLLON, T., and HAUGHTON, E. (1964). Modification of symptomatic verbal behavior of mental patients. *Behavior Research and Therapy*, 2:87-97.

AYLLON, T., and AZRIN, N. H. (1965). The measurement and reinforcement of behavior of psychotics, *Journal of the Experimental Analysis of Behavior*, 8:357-383.

AYLLON, T., and AZRIN, N. H. (1968). The Token Economy: A Motivational System for Therapy and Rehabilitation. New York: Appleton-Century-Crofts.

AYLLON, T., and ROBERTS, M. D. (1972). The token economy now. In *Behavior Modification: Principles and Clinical Applications*, ed. W. S. Agras, Boston: Little, Brown and Co.

BACHMAN, B. (1971). Re-entering the community: a former patient's view. *Hospital and Community Psychiatry*, 22:35-38.

BAER, D. M., WOLF, M. M., and RISLEY, T. R. (1968). Some current dimensions of applied behavior analysis. *Journal of Applied Behavior Analysis*, 1:91-97.

BAILEY, D. M. (1968). A work program in psychiatry. *American Journal of Occupational Therapy*, 22:311-318.

BALL, T. S. (1968). Issues and implications of operant conditioning: the reestablishment of social behavior. *Hospital and Community Psychiatry*, 19:230-232.

BAN, T. (1969). Psychopharmacology. Baltimore: Williams and Wilkins.

BANDURA, A. (1969). Principles of Behavior Modification. New York: Holt, Rinehart and Winston.

BEELS, C. C., and FERBER, A. (1969). Family therapy: a view. *Family Process*, 8:280-318.

BELKNAP, I. (1956). Human Problems of a State Mental Hospital. New York: McGraw-Hill.

BERMAN, K. (1972). Multiple family therapy: its possibilities in preventing readmission. In *Family Therapy: An Introduction to Theory and Practice*, eds. G. D. Erickson and T. P. Hogan, Monterey, Calif.: Brooks/Cole.

BERMAN, L. H. (1972a). Dealing with problems of the therapeutic community. *American Journal of Psychiatry*, 128:1317.

BERMAN, L. H. (1972b). Participation of patients in a psychiatric hospital. A paper presented at the Eastern Psychiatric Research Association, Inc., Third Annual Multistate Interhospital Conference, New York.

BERNE, E. (1966). Principles of Group Treatment. New York: Oxford University Press.

BERNSTEIN, R. E. H., and MASON, P. (1966). Effects of phenothiazine discontinuation in patients compensated from acute psychosis. *Journal of the Mount Sinai Hospital*, 33:131-139.

BERTALANFFY, L. v. (1968). General System Theory: Foundations, Development, Applications. New York: Braziller.

BIJOU, S. W., PETERSON, R. F., and AULT, M. H. (1968). A method to integrate descriptive and experimental field studies at the level of data and empirical concepts. *Journal of Applied Behavior Analysis*, 1:175-191.

BION, W. R. (1961). Experiences in Groups. London: Tavistock.

BOCKOVEN, J. S. (1957). Some relationships between cultural attitudes toward individuality in the care of the mentally ill: a historical study. In *The Patient and the Mental Hospital*, eds. M. Greenblatt, D. J. Levinson, and R. H. Williams, Glencoe, Ill.: Free Press.

BOCKOVEN, J. S. (1963). Moral Treatment in American Psychiatry. New York: Springer.

BODIN, A. M. (1968). Conjoint family assessment: an evolving field. In *Advances in Psychological Assessment*, ed. P. McReynolds, Palo Alto: Science and Behavior Books.

BOWEN, M. (1965). Family psychotherapy with schizophrenia in the hospital and in private practice. In *Intensive Family Therapy*, eds. I. Boszormenyi-Nagy and J. L. Framo, New York: Hoeber, Harper, and Row.

BRADFORD, L. P., GIBB, J. R., and BENNE, K. D. (1964). T-group Therapy and Laboratory Method: Innovation and Re-education. New York: Wiley.

BRAGG, R.A., and WAGNER, M. K. (1968). Issues and implications of operant conditioning: can deprivation be justified? *Hospital and Community Psychiatry*, 19:229-230.

CAFFEY, E. M., GALBRECHT, C. R., and KLETT, C. J. (1971). Brief hospitalization and aftercare in the treatment of schizophrenia. *Archives of General Psychiatry*, 24:81-86.

CAHOON, D. D. (1968). Issues and implications of operant conditioning: balancing procedures against outcome. *Hospital and Community Psychiatry*, 19:228-229.

CAMPBELL, J. P., and DUNNETTE, M. D. (1968). Effectiveness of T-group experiences in managerial training and development. *Psychological Bulletin*, 70:73-104.

CAPLAN, G. (1964). Principles of Preventive Psychiatry. New York: Basic Books.

CARLSON, C. G., HERSEN, M., and EISLER, R. M. (1972). Token economy programs in the treatment of hospitalized adult psychiatric patients. *Journal of Nervous and Mental Disease*, 155:192-204.

CAUDILL, W. (1958). The Psychiatric Hospital as a Small Society. Cambridge: Harvard University Press.

CHIEN, C.-P., and COLE, J. O. (1973). Landlord-supervised cooperative apartments: a new modality for community-based treatment. *American Journal of Psychiatry*, 1:30-156-159.

CLARK, O. E. (1971). Hospital psychiatry—a historical perspective. Unpublished.

CLAUSEN, J. A., and YARROW, M. R. (1955). Paths to the mental hospital. *Journal of Social Issues,* 11 (4):25-32.

COCKRILL, V. K., and BERNAL, M. E. (1968). Operant conditioning of verbal behavior in a withdrawn patient by a patient-peer. *Perspectives in Psychiatric Care,* 6:230-237.

COMMISSION ON LUNACY (1855). Report on Insanity and Idiocy in Massachusetts. Boston: William White.

COTTER, L. H. (1967). Operant conditioning in a Vietnamese mental hospital. *American Journal of Psychiatry,* 134:23-28.

CRABTREE, L. H., and COX, J. L. D. (1972). The overthrow of a therapeutic community. *International Journal of Group Psychotherapy,* 22:31-41.

CURRAY, A. E. (1965). Therapeutic management of multiple family groups. *International Journal of Group Psychotherapy,* 15:90-96.

DAVIES, R. K., and COUGHLAN, P. M. (1970). A conceptualization of individual psychotherapy in a hospital milieu setting. Unpublished.

Department of Health Education, and Welfare (1972). Health Services and Mental Health Administration. Statistical Note 58, Chevy Chase, Md.: National Institute of Mental Health.

DETRE, T., KESSLER, D. R., and SAYERS, J. (1961a). A socio-adaptive approach to treatment of acutely disturbed psychiatric inpatients. *Proceedings of the Third World Congress of Psychiatry,* 1:501-506.

DETRE, T., SAYERS, J., NORTON, N. M., and LEWIS, H. C. (1961b). An experimental approach to the treatment of the acutely ill psychiatric patient in the general hospital. *Connecticut Medicine,* 25:613-619.

DETRE, T., and JARECKI, H. (1971a). Modern Psychiatric Treatment. Philadelphia: Lippincott.

DETRE, T., and TUCKER, G. (1971b). Psychotherapy for the mentally ill: a redefinition of goals. In *The New Hospital Psychiatry,* eds. G. M. Abroms and N. S. Greenfield, New York: Academic.

DEUTSCH, A. (1948). The Shame of the States. New York: Harcourt, Brace.

DEUTSCH, A. (1949). The Mentally Ill in America. New York: Columbia University Press.

DEWALD, P. A. (1964). Psychotherapy: A Dynamic Approach. New York: Basic Books.

DIMASCIO, A. (1970). Dosage scheduling. In *Clinical Handbook of Psychopharmacology,* eds. A. DiMascio and R. I. Shader, New York: Science House.

DIMASCIO, A., and SHADER, R. I. (eds.) (1970b). Clinical Handbook of Psychopharmacology, New York: Science House.

EDELSON, M. (1969). Sociotherapy and psychotherapy in the psychiatric hospital. *Social Psychiatry,* 47:196-211.

ELBERT, S., ROSMAN, B., MINUCHIN, S., and GUERNEY, B. (1964). A method for the clinical study of family interaction. *American Journal of Orthopsychiatry,* 34:885-894.

ENDICOTT, J., and SPITZER, R. L. (1972). Current and past psychopathology scales (CAPS). *Archives of General Psychiatry,* 27:678-687.

ENGLE, R. P., and SEMRAD, E. V. (1971). Brief hospitalization: the recompensation process. In *The New Hospital Psychiatry,* eds. G. M. Abroms and N. S. Greenfield, New York: Academic.

ENGELHARDT, D. M. (1967). Drug treatment of chronic ambulatory patients. *American Journal of Psychiatry,* 123:1329-1337.

ERICKSON, G. D., and HOGAN, T. P. (eds.) (1972). Family Therapy: An Introduction to Theory and Technique. Monterey, Calif.: Brooks/Cole.

FAIRWEATHER, G. W. (ed.) (1964). Social Psychology in Treating Mental Illness: An Experimental Approach. New York: Wiley.

FAIRWEATHER, G. W. (1967). Methods for Experimental Social Innovation. New York: Wiley.

FERSTER, C. B. (1967). Arbitrary and natural reinforcement. Psychological Record, 17:341-347.

FERSTER, C. B. (1971). The use of learning principles in clinical practice and training. Psychological Record, 21:353-361.

FIDLER, G. S., and FIDLER, J. W. (1963). Occupational Therapy: A Communication Process in Psychiatry. New York: Macmillan.

FISCHER, A., and WEINSTEIN, M. R. (1971). Mental hospitals, prestige, and image of enlightenment. Archives of General Psychiatry, 25:41-48.

FORREST, F. M., and FORREST, I. S. (1957). A simple test for the detection of chlorpromazine in urine. American Journal of Psychiatry, 133:913-932.

FORREST, F. M., FORREST, I. S., and MASON, A. S. (1958). A rapid urinary test for chlorpromazine, promazine and pacatal: a supplementary report. American Journal of Psychiatry, 114:931-932.

FORREST, F. M., FORREST, I. S., and MASON, A. S. (1961). Review of rapid urine tests for phenothiazine and related drugs. American Journal of Psychiatry, 118:300-307.

FORREST, F. M., GEITER, C. W., and SNOW, H. L. (1964). Drug maintenance problems of rehabilitated mental patients: the current drug dosage "merry-go-round". American Journal of Psychiatry, 121:33-40.

FORREST, I., and FORREST, F. (1960a). Urine color test for the detection of phenothiazine compounds. Clinical Chemistry, 6:11-15.

FORREST, I. S., FORREST, F.M., and MASON, A. S. (1960b). A rapid urine color test for thioridazine (Mellaril, tp 21, Sandoz). American Journal of Psychiatry, 116:928-929.

FOX, J. V., and JIRGAL, D. (1967). Therapeutic properties of activities as examined by the clinical council of the Wisconsin schools of occupational therapy. American Journal of Occupational Therapy, 21:29-33.

FRANKS, C. M. (ed.). Behavior Therapy: Appraisal and Status. New York: McGraw-Hill.

GARBER, B. (1972). Follow-up Study of Hospitalized Adolescents. New York: Brunner/Mazel.

GARDNER, J. M. (1972). Teaching behavior modification to nonprofessionals. Journal of Applied Behavior Analysis, 5:517-521.

GARLINGTON, W. K., and LLOYD, K. E. (1972). The establishment of a token economy ward at the state hospital north in Orofino, Idaho. A paper presented at Fort Steilacoon, Washington.

GELFAND, D. M., GELFAND, S., and DOBSON, W. R. (1967). Unprogrammed reinforcement of patients' behavior in a mental hospital. Behavior Research and Therapy, 5:201-207.

GERICKE, O. L. (1965). Practical use of operant conditioning procedures in a mental hospital. Psychiatric Studies and Projects, 3:2-10.

GOFFMAN, E. (1961). Asylums: Essays on the Social Situation of Mental Patients and Other Inmates. Garden City, N. J.: Doubleday.

GONEN, J. Y. (1971). The use of psychodrama combined with videotape playback on an inpatient floor. Psychiatry, 34:198-213.

GORHAM, D. R., and POKORNY, A. D. (1964). Effects of a phenothiazine and/or group psychotherapy with schizophrenics. *Diseases of the Nervous System,* 25:77-86.

GOVE, W. R., and FAIN, T. (1973). The stigma of mental hospitalization. *Archives of General Psychiatry,* 28:494-500.

GRALNICK, A. (1969a). The Psychiatric Hospital as a Therapeutic Instrument. New York: Brunner/Mazel.

GRALNICK, A., and D'ELIA, F. (1969b). A psychoanalytic hospital becomes a therapeutic community. *Hospital and Community Psychiatry,* 20:144-146.

GRANT, R. L., and SASLOW, G. (1971). Maximizing responsible decision making, or how to get out of here? In *The New Hospital Psychiatry,* eds. G. B. Abroms and N. S. Greenfield, New York: Academic.

GRANT, R. L., and MALETZKY, B. M. (1972). Application of the Weed system to psychiatric records. *Psychiatry in Medicine,* 3:119-129.

GREENBLATT, M., YORK, R. H., and BROWN, E. C. (1955). From Custodial to Therapeutic Patient Care in Mental Hospitals. New York: Russell Sage Foundation.

GREENBLATT, M., MOORE, R. F., ALBERT, R. S., and SOLOMON, N. H. (1963). The Prevention of Hospitalization: Treatment Without Admission for Psychiatric Patients. New York: Grune and Stratton.

GREENLEY, J. R. (1973). Power processes and patient behaviors. *Archives of General Psychiatry,* 28:683-688.

GRINSPOON, L., EWALT, J. R., and SHADER, R. (1967). Long-term treatment of chronic schizophrenia: a preliminary report. *International Journal of Psychiatry,* 4:116-128.

Group for the Advancement of Psychiatry (1969). Crisis in psychiatric hospitalization. No. 72, 7:64-71.

GRUENBERG, E. M. (1967). The social breakdown syndrome—some origins. *American Journal of Psychiatry,* 123:1481-1489.

GUY, W., and BONATO, R. R. (1970). Manual for the ECDEU Assessment Battery. Chevy Chase, Md.: National Institute of Mental Health.

HADEN, P. (1959). Drugs—single or multiple daily dosage? *American Journal of Psychiatry,* 115:932-933.

HALL, R. V. (1970a). Behavior Management Series—Part I. Behavior Modification: The Measurement of Behavior. Marriam, Kansas: H and H Enterprises.

HALL, R. V., CRISTLER, C., CRANSTON, S. S., and TUCKER, B. (1970b). Teachers and parents as researchers using multiple baseline designs. *Journal of Applied Behavior Analysis,* 3:247-255.

HAMILTON, S. W. (1944). The history of American mental hospitals. In *One Hundred Years of American Psychiatry,* ed. J. K. Hall, New York: Columbia University Press.

HANSEN, P. G., ROTHAUS, P., JOHNSON, D. L., and LYLE, F. A. (1964). Autonomous groups in human relations training for psychiatric patients. Paper presented at the annual meeting of the American Psychological Association, Los Angeles

HARE, E. H., and WILLCOX, D. R. C. (1967). Do psychiatric inpatients take their pills? *British Journal of Psychiatry,* 113:1435-1439.

HARROW, M., ASTRACHAN, B. M., BECKER, R. E., DETRE, T., and SCHWARTZ, A. H. (1967). An investigation into the nature of the patient-family therapy group. *American Journal of Orthopsychiatry,* 37:888-899.

HARROW, M., FOX, D. A., MARKHUS, K. L., STILLMAN, R., and HALLOWELL, C. B. (1968). Changes in adolescents' self-concepts and their parents' perceptions during psychiatric hospitalization. *Journal of Nervous and Mental Disease,* 147:252-259.

HARROW, M., FOX, D. A., and DETRE, T. (1969). Self-concept of the married psychiatric patient and his mate's perception of him. *Journal of Consulting and Clinical Psychology*, 33:235-239.

HARROW, M., TUCKER, G. J., and SHIELD, P. (1972). Stimulus overinclusion and schizophrenic disorders. *Archives of General Psychiatry*, 27:40-45.

HAUN, P. (1971). Recreation: A Medical Viewpoint, New York: Teacher's College.

HAVENS, L. L. (1963). Problems with the use of drugs in the psychotherapy of psychotic patients. *Psychiatry*, 26:289-296.

HAVENS, L. L. (1968). Some difficulties in giving schizophrenic and borderline patients medication. *Psychiatry*, 31:44-50.

HAVENS, L. L. (1970). Interaction of drug administration with psychotherapy. In *Clinical Handbook of Psychopharmacology*, eds. A. DiMascio and R. I. Shader, New York: Science House.

HENDERSON, D., and GILLESPIE, R. D. (1952). A Textbook of Psychiatry for Students and Practitioners. London: Oxford University Press.

HENDERSON, J. D., and SCOLES, P. E., Jr. (1970). Conditioning techniques in a community-based operant environment for psychotic men. *Behavior Therapy*, 1:245-251.

HERSEN, M., EISLER, R. M., SMITH, B. S., and AGRAS, W. S. (1972). A token reinforcement ward for young psychiatric patients. *American Journal of Psychiatry*, 129: 228-233

HERZ, M. I., ENDICOTT, J., SPITZER, R. L., and MESNIKOFF, A. (1971). Day versus inpatient hospitalization: a controlled study. *American Journal of Psychiatry*, 127:1371-1382.

HERZ, M. I. (1972). The therapeutic community: a critique. *Hospital and Community Psychiatry*, 23:69-72.

HES, J. P., and HANDLER, S. L. (1961). Multidimensional group psychotherapy. *Archives of General Psychiatry*, 5:70-75.

HILLES, L. (1970). Critical incidents precipitating admissions to a psychiatric hospital. *Bulletin of the Menninger Clinic*, 34:89-102.

HOGARTY, G. E., and ULRICH, R. (1972). The discharge readiness inventory. *Archives of General Psychiatry*, 26:419-426.

HOLLINGSHEAD, A. B., and REDLICH, F. C. (1958). Social Class and Mental Illness: A Community Study. New York: Wiley.

HOUPT, J. L., ASTRACHAN, B., LIPSITCH, I., and ANDERSON, C. (1972). Re-entry groups: bridging the hospital-community gap. *Social Psychiatry*, 7:144-149.

IMBODEN, J. B., UNGER, H. T., and MARKEY, R. B. (1965). Inpatient service at the Henry Phipps psychiatric clinic. In *Current Psychiatric Therapies*, ed. J. Masserman, New York: Grune and Stratton, 5:218-222.

IRWIN, D. S., WEITZEL, W. D., and MORGAN, D. W. (1971). Phenothiazine intake and staff attitudes. *American Journal of Psychiatry*, 127:1631-1635.

JACOBS, A., and SACHS, L. (eds.) (1971). The Psychology of Private Events. New York: Academic.

JOHNSON, C. A., KATZ, R. C., and GELFAND, S. (1972). Undergraduates as behavioral technicians on an adult token economy ward. *Behavior Therapy*, 3:589-592.

JOHNSON, S. M., and BOLSTEAD, O. D. (1973). Methodological issues in naturalistic observation: some problems and solutions for field research. In *Behavior Change: Methodology Concepts and Practice*, eds., L. A. Hamerlynck, L. C. Handy, and E. J. Mash, Champaign, Ill.: Research Press.

JONES, M. (1953). The Therapeutic Community: A New Treatment Method in Psychiatry. New York: Basic Books.

JONES, M. (1965). A passing glance at the therapeutic community in 1964. *International Journal of Group Psychotherapy*, 15:5-10.

JONES, M. (1968). Beyond the Therapeutic Community: Social Learning and Social Psychiatry. New Haven: Yale University.

JONES, N. F., KAHN, M. W., and LANGSLEY, D. G. (1965). Prediction of admission to a psychiatric hospital. *Archives of General Psychiatry*, 12:607-610.

JOURNAL OF THE AMERICAN HOSPITAL ASSOCIATION. (1971). The nation's hospitals: a statistical profile. 45:447-489.

KADIS, A. L. (1956). The alternate meeting and group psychotherapy. *American Journal of Psychotherapy*, 10:275-291.

KALOGERAKIS, M. G. (1971). The assaultive psychiatric patient. *Psychiatric Quarterly*, 45:372-381.

KATZ, R. C., JOHNSON, C. A., and GELFAND, S. (1972). Modifying the dispensing of reinforcers: some implications for behavior modification with hospitalized patients. *Behavior Therapy*, 3:579-588.

KAZDIN, A. E. (1972a). Nonresponsiveness of patients to token economies. *Behaviour Research and Therapy*, 10:417-418.

KAZDIN, A. E., and BOOTZIN, R. R. (1972b). The token economy: an evaluative review. *Journal of Applied Behavior Analysis*, 5:343-372.

KERNBERG, O. F. (1973). Discussion of G. Adler: Hospital treatment of borderline patients. *American Journal of Psychiatry*, 130:32-36.

KLEIN, D. F., and DAVIS, J. N. (1969). Diagnosis and Drug Treatment of Psychiatric Disorders. Baltimore: Williams and Wilkins.

KOLE, C., and DANIELS, R. S. (1966). An operational model for a therapeutic community. *International Journal of Group Psychotherapy*, 16:279-290.

KRAMER, J. C. (1962). Single daily dose schedules of imipramine (Tofranil). *Comprehensive Psychiatry*, 3:191-192.

KRAUS, R. (1972). Recreation and related therapies in psychiatric rehabilitation: a research study. Unpublished.

KUBIE, L. S. (1960). The Riggs Story: The Development of the Austin Riggs Center for the Study and Treatment of the Neuroses. New York: Hoeber.

KUPFER, D. J., and DETRE, T. P. (1971a). Commentary: once more—on the extraordinary side effects of drugs. *Clinical Pharmacology and Therapeutics*, 12:575-582.

KUPFER, D. J., and DETRE, T. P. (1971b). KDS^{tm} Systems, Inc. Woodbridge, Conn.: KDS Systems, Inc.

LAING, R. D. (1967). The Politics of Experience. New York: Pantheon.

LAMB, H. R., and GOERTZEL, V. (1971). Discharged mental patients—are they really in the community? *Archives of General Psychiatry*, 24:29-34.

LANGSLEY, D. G., MACHOTKA, P., and FLOMENHAFT, K. (1971). Avoiding mental hospital admission: a follow-up study. *American Journal of Psychiatry*, 127:1391-1394.

LAQUER, H. P., LaBURT, H. A., and MORONG, E. (1964). Multiple family therapy. In Current Psychiatric Therapies, ed. J. Masserman, New York: Grune and Stratton, 4:150-154.

LAZARE, A., COHEN, F., JACOBSEN, A., WILLIAMS, M. W., MIGNONE, R., and ZISOOK, S. (1972). The walk-in patient as a 'consumer': a key to evaluation and treatment. *American Journal of Orthopsychiatry*, 42:872-883.

LeBow, M. D. (1972). Behavior modification for the family. In *Family Therapy: An Introduction to Theory and Technique*, eds. G. D. Erickson and T. P. Hogan, Monterey, Calif.: Brooks/Cole.

LeBow, M. D. (1973). Behavior Modification: A Significant Method in Nursing Practice. Englewood Cliffs, N. J.: Prentice-Hall.

LEHMANN, H. E. (1970). Interaction of pharmacotherapy with total treatment. In *Clinical Handbook of Psychopharmacology*, eds. A. DiMascio and R. I. Shader, New York: Science House.

LEITENBERG, H. W., AGRAS, W. S., and THOMSON, L. (1968). A sequential analysis of the effect of selective positive reinforcement in modifying anorexia nervosa. *Behaviour Research and Therapy*, 6:211-218.

LEVIN, E. C. (1966). Therapeutic multiple family groups. *International Journal of Group Psychotherapy*, 16:203-208.

LEWIS, F. A. (1962). Community care of psychiatric patients versus prolonged institutionalization. *Journal of the American Medical Association*, 182:323-326.

LEWIS, J. C., and GLASSER, N. (1965). Evaluation of a treatment approach to families: group family therapy. *International Journal of Group Psychotherapy*, 15: 505-515.

LIBERMAN, R. (1970). Behavioral approaches to family and couple therapy. *American Journal of Orthopsychiatry*, 40:106-118.

LICHTENBERG, J. B., and PAO, P.-N. (1960). The prognostic and therapeutic significance of the husband-wife relationship for hospitalized schizophrenic women. *Psychiatry*, 23: 209-213.

LIDZ, T., PARKER, B., and CORNELISON, A. (1956). The role of the father in the family environment of the schizophrenic patient. *American Journal of Psychiatry*, 113: 126-132.

LIEB, J., LIPSITCH, I. I., and SLABY, A. E. (1973). The Crisis Team: A Handbook for the Mental Health Professional. Hagerstown, Md.: Harper and Row.

LINDEMANN, E. (1944). Symptomatology and management of acute grief. *American Journal of Psychiatry*, 101:141-148.

LINDSLEY, O. R., and SKINNER, B. F. (1954). A method for the experimental analysis of the behavior of psychotic patients. *American Psychologist*, 9:419-420.

LINN, E. L. (1960). The association of preadmission symptoms with the social background of mental patients. *Archives of General Psychiatry*, 8:557-562.

LINN, L. (1955). A Handbook of Hospital Psychiatry: A Practical Guide to Therapy. New York: International Universities Press.

LINN, L. S. (1968). The mental hospital from the patient perspective. *Psychiatry*, 31:213-223.

LINN, L. S. (1969). Social characteristics and patient expectations toward mental hospitalization. *Archives of General Psychiatry*, 20:457-469.

LION, J. R., and PASTERNAK, S. A. (1973) Countertransference reactions to violent patients. *American Journal of Psychiatry*, 130:207-210.

LIPSIUS, L. H. (1973). The Weed system and psychiatry. *American Journal of Psychiatry*, 130:610-611.

LLOYD, K. E., and ABEL, L. (1970). Performance on a token economy psychiatric ward: a two year summary. *Behaviour Research and Therapy*, 8:1-9.

LORR, M., McNAIR, D. M., KLETT, C. J., and LASKY, J. J. (1962) Evidence of ten psychotic syndromes. *Journal of Consulting Psychology*, 26:185-189.

LUCERO, R. J., VAIL, D. J., and SCHERBER, J. (1968). Regulating operant-conditioning programs. *Hospital and Community Psychiatry*, 19:53-54.

LUDWIG, A. M., and FARRELLY, F. (1966). The code of chronicity. *Archives of General Psychiatry*, 15:562-568.

LUDWIG, A. M. (1971). Responsibility and chronicity: new treatment models for the chronic schizophrenic. In *The New Hospital Psychiatry*, eds. G. M. Abroms and N. S. Greenfield, New York: Academic.

MACDONALD, J. M. (1965). "Acting-out". *Archives of General Psychiatry*, 13:439-442.

MACDONALD, J. M. (1966). The prompt diagnosis of psychopathic personality. *American Journal of Psychiatry*, 122 (June supplement) : 45-50.

MAIN, T. F. (1957). The ailment. *British Journal of Medical Psychology*, 30:129-145.

MALAMUD, W. (1944). The history of psychiatric therapies. In *One Hundred Years of American Psychiatry*, ed. J. K. Hall, New York: Columbia University Press.

MAROHN, R. C., DALLE-MOLLE, D., OFFER, D., and OSTROV, E. (1973). A hospital riot: its determinants and implications for treatment. *American Journal of Psychiatry*, 130:631-636.

MAXMEN, J. S. (1973a). Group therapy as viewed by hospitalized patients. *Archives of General Psychiatry*, 28: 404-408.

MAXMEN, J. S., and TUCKER, G. J. (1973b). The admission process. *Journal of Nervous and Mental Disease*, 156:327-340.

MAXMEN, J. S., and TUCKER, G. J. (1973c). No exist: the persistently suicidal patient. *Comprehensive Psychiatry*, 14:71-79.

MAY, P. R. A., and TUMA, A. H. (1964). The effect of psychotherapy and Stelazine on length of hospital stay, release rate and supplemental treatment of schizophrenic patients. *Journal of Nervous and Mental Disease,* 139:362-369.

MENDEL, W. M. (1968). On the abolition of the psychiatric hosiptal. In *Comprehensive Mental Health*, eds. L. M. Roberts, N. S. Greenfield, and M. H. Miller, Madison, Wis.: University of Wisconsin.

MENDEL, W. M., and RAPPORT, S. (1969). Determinants of the decision for psychiatric hospitalization. *Archives of General Psychiatry*, 20:321-328.

MENNINGER, W. (1936). Psychoanalytic principles applied to the treatment of hospitalized patients. *Bulletin of the Menninger Clinic*, 1:35-43.

MILLER, E. J. and RICE, A. K. (1967). Systems of Organization: The Control of Task and Sentient Boundaries. London: Tavistock.

MINUCHIN, S., MONTALVO, B., GUERNEY, B. G. ROSMAN, B. L., and SCHUMER, F. (1967). Families of the Slums: An Exploration of Their Structure and Treatment. New York: Basic Books.

MIRON, N. B. (1968). Issues and implications of operant conditioning: the primary ethical consideration. *Hospital and Community Psychiatry*, 19:226-228.

MITCHELL, S. W. (1894). Fiftieth anniversary address. Transactions of the American Medico-Psychological Association.

MOOS, R. H. (1967). Differential effects of ward settings on psychiatric patients. *Journal of Nervous and Mental Disease*, 145:272-283.

MOOS, R. H. (1968). Differential effects of ward settings on psychiatric patients: a replication and extension. *Journal of Nervous and Mental Disease*, 147:386-393.

MORENO, J. L. (1959). Psychodrama. In *American Handbook of Psychiatry*, ed. S. Arieti, Volume 2, New York: Basic Books.

MORENO, J. L. (1966). Therapeutic aspects of psychodrama. *Psychiatric Opinion*, 3 (2) :36-42.

MOSEY, A. C. (1970). Three Frames of Reference for Mental Health. Thorofare, N. J.: Charles B. Slack.

MULLER, D. J. (1971). Post-camping depression: a lethal possibility. *American Journal of Psychiatry*, 128:141-143.

MULLER, J. J., CHAFETZ, M. E., and BLANE, H. T. (1967). Acute psychiatric services in the general hospital: III statistical survey. *American Journal of Psychiatry*, 124 (supplement) : 46-57.

MYERS, K., and CLARK, D. H. (1972). Results in a therapeutic community. *British Journal of Psychiatry*, 120:51-58.

NEVE, H. K. (1958). Demonstration of Largactil (chlorpromazine hydrochloride) in the urine. *Journal of Mental Science*, 104:488-490.

NEW YORK TIMES. (1972). July 30, p. 36.

NORTON, N. M., DETRE, T. P., and JARECKI, H. G. (1963). Psychiatric services in general hospitals: a family-oriented redefinition. *Journal of Nervous and Mental Disease*, 136:475-484.

O'BRIEN, F., and AZRIN, N. H. (1973). Interaction-priming: a method of reinstating patient-family relationships. *Behaviour Research and Therapy*, 11:133-136.

OVERALL, J. E., and GORHAM, D. R. (1962). The brief psychiatric rating scale. *Psychological Report*, 10:799-812.

PANYAN, M., BOOZER, H., and MORRIS, N. (1970). Feedback to attendants as a reinforcer for applying operant techniques. *Journal of Applied Behavior Analysis*, 3:1-4.

PAO, P.-N. (1960). The use of patient-family doctor interviews to facilitate the schizophrenic patient's return to the community. *Psychiatry*, 23:199-207.

PASAMANICK, B., SCARPITTI, F. R., and DINITZ, S. (1967). Schizophrenics in the Community: An Experimental Study in the Prevention of Hospitalization. New York: Appleton-Century-Crofts.

PATTERSON, G. R., COBB, J., and RAY, R. A. (1970a). A social engineering technology for retraining aggressive boys. In *Georgia Symposium in Experimental Clinical Psychology*, eds. H. Adams and L. Unikel, New York: Pergamon.

PATTERSON, G. R., and REID, J. B. (1970b). Reciprocity and coercion: two facets of social systems. In *Behavior Modification in Clinical Psychology*, eds. C. Neuringer and J. Michael, New York: Appleton-Century-Crofts.

PAUL, G. L. (1969). Chronic mental patient: current status-future direction. *Psychological Bulletin*, 71:81-94.

PETERSON, D. P., and OLSEN, G. W. (1963). Single- versus multiple-dose administration of tranquilizing medications. *Psychiatric Studies and Projects*, 14:2-4.

PIERCE, W. D., TRICKETT, E. J., and MOOS, R. H. (1972). Changing ward atmosphere through staff discussion of the perceived ward environment. *Archives of General Psychiatry*, 26:35-41.

PINSKER, H. (1966). Fallacies in hospital community therapy. In *Current Psychiatric Therapies*, ed. J. Masserman, New York: Grune and Stratton, 6:344-352.

POLAK, P., and LAYCOB, L. (1971). Rapid tranquilization. *American Journal of Psychiatry*, 128:640-643.

POLANSKY, N. A., and HARKINS, E. B. (1969). Psychodrama as an element in hospital treatment. *Psychiatry*, 32:74-87.

POSER, E. G. (1972). Training behavior change agents: a five year perspective. In *Implementing Behavioral Programs for Schools and Clinics. Proceedings of the Third Banff International Conference on Behavior Modification*, eds. F. W. Clark, D. R. Evans, L. A. Hamerlynck, Champaign, Ill.: Research Press.

PRATT, J. H. (1906). The home sanatorium treatment of consumption. *Bulletin of the Johns Hopkins Hospital*, 17:140-158.

PREMACK, D. (1959). Toward empirical behavioral laws: I. positive reinforcement. *Psychological Review,* 66:219-233.

PREMACK, D. (1963). Prediction of the comparative reinforcement values of running and drinking. *Science,* 139:1062-1063.

QUERIDO, A. (1965). Early Diagnosis and Treatment Services in Elements of a Community Mental Health Program. Millbank Memorial Fund, Inc.

RASKIN, D. E. (1971). Problems in the therapeutic community. *American Journal of Psychiatry,* 128:492-493.

REDLICH, F. C., and ASTRACHAN, B. M. (1969). Group dynamics training. *American Journal of Psychiatry,* 125:1501-1507.

Report of the Commissioners Appointed to Superintend the Erection of a Lunatic Hospital in Worcester (1832) Massachusetts Documents, no. 2.

REYNOLDS, G. S. (1968). A Primer of Operant Conditioning. Glenview, Ill.: Foresman.

RICE, A. K. (1965). Learning for Leadership. London, Tavistock.

RINSLEY, D. B. (1968). Theory and practice of intensive residential treatment of adolescents. *Psychiatric Quarterly,* 42:611-638.

ROGOFF, M.-L., SUDDUTH, D., and LITTLEWOOD, J. (1973). Group therapy information. Unpublished.

ROSENBERG, S. D. (1970). The disculturation hypothesis and the chronic patient syndrome. *Social Psychiatry,* 5:155-165.

ROSENZWEIG, N. (1967). Planning a psychiatric program for the general hospital. *Hospitals,* 41 (1):58-65.

ROTHAUS, P., JOHNSON, D. L., HANSON, P. G., and LYLE, F. A. (1964) Autonomous and trainer-led patient groups. Paper presented at the annual meeting of the American Psychological Association, Los Angeles.

ROTHMAN, D. J., (1971). The Discovery of the Asylum: Social Order and Disorder in the New Republic. Boston: Little, Brown, and Co.

RUBENSTEIN, R., and LASSWELL, H. D. (1966). The Sharing of Power in a Psychiatric Hospital. New Haven, Yale University.

SADOFF, R. L., ROETHER, H. A., and PETERS, J. J. (1971). Clinical measure of enforced group psychotherapy. *American Journal of Psychiatry,* 128:224-227.

SAGER, C. J. (1972a). Staff development for a therapeutic community. In *Progress in Group and Family Therapy,* eds. C. J. Sager and H. S. Kaplan, New York: Brunner/Mazel.

SAGER, C. J., and KAPLAN, H. S. (eds.) (1972b). Progress in Group and Family Therapy. New York: Brunner/Mazel.

SANDERS, D. H. (1973). Aftercare for discharged patients. A panel presented at the annual meeting of the American Orthopsychiatric Association, New York.

SARWER-FONER, G. J. (1970). Psychodynamics of psychotropic medication—an overview. In *Clinical Handbook of Psychopharmacology,* eds. A. DiMascio and R. I. Shader, New York: Science House.

SCHAEFER, H. H., and MARTIN, P. L. (1966). Behavioral therapy for "apathy" of hospitalized schizophrenics. *Psychological Reports,* 19:1147-1158.

SCHAEFER, H. H., and MARTIN, P. L. (1969). *Behavioral Therapy.* New York: McGraw-Hill.

SCHEIN, E H. and BENNIS, W. G. (1965). Personal and Organizational Change Through Group Methods: The Laboratory Approach. New York: Wiley.

SCHULBERG, H., and SHELDON, A. (1968). The probability of crisis and strategies for for preventive intervention. *Archives of General Psychiatry,* 18:553-558.

SHANFIELD, S., TUCKER, G. J., HARROW, M., and DETRE, T. (1970). The schizophrenic patient and depressive symptomatology. *Journal of Nervous and Mental Disease*, 151:203-210

SHERMAN, J. A., and BAER, D. M. (1969). Appraisal of operant therapy techniques with children and adults. In *Behavior Therapy: Appraisal and Status*, ed. C. M. Franks, New York: McGraw-Hill.

SKINNER, B. F. (1938). The Behavior of Organisms. New York: Appleton-Century-Crofts.

SKINNER, B. F. (1953). Science and Human Behavior. New York: Macmillan.

SKINNER, B. F. (1969). Contingencies of Reinforcement: A Theoretical Analysis. New York: Appleton-Century-Crofts.

SLAVSON, S. R. (1964). A Textbook in Analytic Group Psychotherapy. New York: International Universities Press.

SMITH, C. G. and SINANAN, K. (1972). The "gaslight phenomenon" reappears: a modification of the Ganser syndrome. *British Journal of Psychiatry*, 120:685-686.

SMITH, R. C., and CARLIN, J. (1972). Behavior modification using interlocking reinforcement on a short-term psychiatric ward. *Archives of General Psychiatry*, 27: 386-389.

SOLOMON, L. N., and BERZON, B. (eds.) (1972). New Perspectives on Encounter Groups. San Francisco: Jossey-Bass.

SOLOW, C., WEISS, R. J., BERGEN, B. J., and SANBORN, C. J. (1971). 24-hour psychiatric consultation via TV. *American Journal of Psychiatry*, 127:1684-1687.

SPADONI, A. J., and SMITH, J. A. (1969). Milieu therapy in schizophrenia: a negative result. *Archives of General Psychiatry*, 20:547-551.

SPITZER, R. L., FLEISS, J. L., KERNOHAN, W., LEE, J. C., and BALDWIN, I. T. (1965). The mental status schedule: comparing Kentucky and New York schizophrenics. *Archives of General Psychiatry*, 12:448-455.

SPITZER, R. L., ENDICOTT, J., FLEISS, J. L., and COHEN, J. (1970). The psychiatric status schedule: a technique for evaluating psychopathology and impairment in role functioning. *Archives of General Psychiatry*, 23:41-55.

STANCER, H. C., SOURS, J. A., and GIDRO-FRANK, L. (1965). Interpersonal psychodynamics of voluntary psychiatry admissions. *Psychiatric Quarterly*, 39:1-21.

STANTON, A. H., and SCHWARTZ, M. S. (1954). The Mental Hospital: A Study of Institutional Participation in Psychiatric Illness and Treatment. New York: Basic Books.

SULLIVAN, H. S. (1931). Socio-psychiatric research: its implication for the schizophrenic problem and for mental hygiene. *American Journal of Psychiatry*, 10: 977-991.

SUTHERLAND, J. D. (1952). Notes on psychoanalytic group therapy: I. therapy and training. *Psychiatry*, 15:111-117.

SZASZ, T. S. (1961). The Myth of Mental Illness. New York: Harper and Row.

THOMAS, C. S., and WEISMAN, G. K. (1970). Emergency planning: the practical and theoretical backdrop to an emergency treatment unit. *International Journal of Social Psychiatry*, 16:283-287.

TUCKER, G. J., and MAXMEN, J. S. (1972). Multiple family group therapy in a psychiatric hospital. *Journal of Psychoanalysis in Groups*, 4 (1):27-34.

TUCKER, G. J., and MAXMEN, J. S. (1973). The practice of hospital psychiatry: a formulation. *American Journal of Psychiatry*, 130:887-891.

UHLENHUTH, E. H., RICKELS, K., FISHER, S., PARK, L. C., LIPMAN, R. S., and MOCK, J. (1966). Drug doctor's verbal attitude and clinic setting in the symptomatic response to pharmacotherapy. *Psychopharmacologia*, 9:392-418.

UNDERWOOD, W. J. (1965). Evaluation of laboratory method training. *Training sponse to pharmacotherapy. Psychopharmacologia, 9:392-418. Directors Journal, 19 (5):34-40.*

UPPER, D. (1971). A "ticket" system for reducing ward rules violations on a token economy program. Paper presented at the annual meeting of the Association for the Advancement of Behavior Therapy.

VAILLANT, G. E. (1964). Prospective prediction of schizophrenic remission. *Archives of General Psychiatry, 11:509-518.*

WACHSPRESS, M. (1965). Use of groups in various modalities of hospital treatment. *International Journal of Group Psychotherapy, 15:17-22.*

WANKLIN, J. M., FLEMING, D. F., BRUCH, C. W., and HOBBS, C. E. (1955). Factors influencing rate of admissions to mental hospitals.. *Journal of Nervous and Mental Disease, 121:103-116.*

WEED, L. L. (1969). Medical Records, Medical Education, and Patient Care. Cleveland: Press of Case Western Reserve University.

WEINTRAUB, W. (1964). "The V.I.P. syndrome": a clinical study in hospital psychiatry. *Journal of Nervous and Mental Disease, 138:181-193.*

WEISMAN, G., FEIRSTEIN, A., and THOMAS, C. (1969). Three-day hospitalization—a model for intensive intervention. *Archives of General Psychiatry, 21:620-629.*

WHITAKER, C. A., and OLSEN, E. (1971). The staff and the family square off. In *The New Hospital Psychiatry*, eds. G. M. Abroms and N. S. Greenfield, New York: Academic Press.

WHITELY, J. S. (1970). The response of psychopaths to a therapeutic community. *British Journal of Psychiatry, 116:517-529.*

WILMER, H. A. (1958a). Social Psychiatry in Action. Springfield, Ill.: Charles C. Thomas.

WILMER, H. A. (1958b). Towards a definition of the therapeutic community. *American Journal of Psychiatry, 114:824-834.*

WINER, B. J. (1962). Statistical Principles in Experimental Design. New York: McGraw-Hill.

WOLF, A. (1949). The psychoanalysis of groups. *American Journal of Psychotherapy, 3:525-558.*

WOLPE, J. (1969). The Practice of Behavior Therapy. New York: Pergamon Press.

WOOD, E. C., RAKUSIN, J. M., and MORSE, E. (1960). Interpersonal aspects of psychiatric hospitalization: I. The admission. *Archives of General Psychiatry. 3:632-641.*

WYNNE, L. C., RYCKOFF, I. M., DAY, J., and HIRSCH, S. I. (1958). Pseudo-mutuality in the family relations of schizophrenics. *Psychiatry, 21:205-220.*

YALOM, I. D. (1970). The Theory and Practice of Group Psychotherapy. New York: Basic Books.

ZEITLYN, B. B. (1967). The therapeutic community—fact or fantasy? *British Journal of Psychiatry, 113:1083-1086.*

INDEX

Abroms, G. M., 29, 38, 40, 45, 58, 76, 119, 127, 147, 193, 230, 261
Ackerman, N. W., 192, 261
Acting-up behavior, 131-135
Activities therapy, 167-176
  abuses of, 173-176
  diagnostic functions of, 168-170
  functions of, 168
  therapeutic functions of, 170-172
Adjustment to community, factors in, 41, 210-212
Admission procedures, 117-125
  criteria for, 120-123
  factors affecting, 118-119
  goals of, 123-125
Advisory board of Tompkins-I 60-62, 70, 75
  by-laws for, 253-256
  constitution of, 245-252
Aftercare preparations, 43, 209-222
  and activities therapy, 172
  and discharge planning groups, 216
  and Discharge Readiness Inventory, 217
  environmental issues in, 210-217
  and extension of hospital programs into home, 213-215
  family participation in, 204-208, 211-215
  historical aspects of, 13
  and home visits by staff, 107, 206-207, 215
  principles of, 210-219
  program in, 219-222
  and referral to outside therapist, 217-219
  and resistance to medications, 164-166
Agras, W. S., 9, 95, 99, 261
Aitchison, R. A., 80, 96, 261
Alexander, F. G., 14, 261
Alienists, role of, 8, 9, 10, 12
Almond, R., 29, 74, 261, 262
Almshouses, confinement in, 6
Apartment living, supervised, 220-221
Astrachan, B. M., 186, 231, 262
Atthowe, J., 97, 262
Attitudes toward hospitalization, 3-5, 19
  of patients, 119-120
Austin Riggs Center, 16
Authority relationships, in therapeutic community, 74-77
Ayd, F., 165, 166, 262
Ayllon, T., 18, 30, 78, 85, 92, 93, 95, 96, 101, 102, 107, 232, 262
Azrin, N. H., 85, 92, 206, 262

Bachman, B., 212, 221, 262
Baer, D. M., 9, 146, 242, 243, 262
Bailey, D. M., 170, 262
Ball, T. S., 110, 111, 262
Ban, T., 151, 262
Bandura, A., 90, 100, 101, 241, 262
Beels, C. C., 198, 262
Behavior
  categories of problems in, 37

concepts of, 85-91, 108-113
as focus of treatment, 36-40
Behavior modification procedures,
103-105
aversive stimulation, 105
demonstration-imitation, 104
extinction, 101-102, 105
instruction, 103
interaction priming, 206-207
negative reinforcement, 87-88,
104
positive reinforcement, 87, 92,
100-101, 103, 147
reinforcing other behavior, 102,
105
response-cost, 102, 105
satiation, 98, 105
shaping, 80, 103
time-out, 105
withdrawal of positive reinforcement, 105
Behavior modification programs,
81-85, 144-149
collecting data in, 91-96, 147-148
for individual patients, 144-149
in therapeutic community, 147
and evaluation, 149, 239-243
historical aspects of, 8-9, 18
See also Reinforcers
See also Token economy
Belknap, I., 4, 262
Berman, K., 201, 202, 204, 262
Berman, L. H., 29, 263
Bernal, M. E., 144, 264
Berne, E., 180, 263
Bernstein, R. E. H., 160, 263
Bertalanffy, L. v., 126, 263
Bijou, S. W., 109, 195, 263
Biological era of hospital psychia-
try, 13-15
Bion, W. R., 178, 180, 263
Bloomingdale Asylum, 8
Bockoven, J. S., 6, 10, 12, 31, 263
Bodin, A. M., 194, 195, 263
Boozer, H., 106 271
Bowen, M., 119, 263
Bradford, L. P., 180, 263
Bragg, R. A., 110, 263

Caffey, E. M., 55, 263
Cahoon, D. D., 110, 111, 263

Campbell, J. P., 229, 263
Caplan, G., 24, 49-50, 263
Carlin, J., 100, 273
Carlson, C. G., 92, 95, 263
Caudill, W., 28, 73, 263
Chestnut Lodge, 16
Chien, C.-P., 221, 263
Clark, O. E., 8, 263
Classification of psychiatric hos-
pitals, 21-32
Clausen, J. A., 118, 264
Cockrill, V. K., 144, 264
Community lodges, 220
Community mental health centers,
development of, 18-19
Confidentiality, in therapeutic com-
munity, 71, 73
Confinement of patients, historical
aspects of, 5-7
Connecticut Mental Health Center,
50-53
Contingencies in behavioral modifi-
cation, 91, 97
Cotter, L. H., 88, 264
Coughlin, P. M., 143, 264
County care plan, versus state care,
11
Cowles, E., 12
Crabtree, L. H., 74, 264
Crisis intervention, 24, 27, 49-55
in Connecticut Mental Health
Center, 50-53
in Dartmouth-Hitchcock Mental
Health Center, 53-55
goals of, 51-52
and outpatient treatment, 55
results of, 52, 54
staff role in, 51, 54
techniques in, 51
Crisis situations, development of,
50
Criticisms of psychiatric hospitals,
3-5, 19
Curray, A. E., 202, 264
Custodial care, 5-7, 26, 30-31

Dartmouth-Hitchcock Mental
Health Center, 53-55, 257
Davies, R. K., 128, 143, 264
Deprivation, as behavior modifier,
110-111

Detre, T., 59, 128, 151, 157, 158, 201, 264
Deutsch, A., 4, 6, 7, 9, 11, 13, 264
Dewald, P. A., 25, 264
DiMascio, A., 151, 162, 166, 264
Discharge Readiness Inventory, 217
Discharged patients. See Aftercare preparations
Discrimination process, in behavior modification, 89-91
Dix, D., 10
Drug therapy. See Medications

Edelson, M., 29, 264
Elbert, S., 195, 264
Electroconvulsive therapy, 14, 26, 30, 156
Emergency sessions, in therapeutic community, 65
Encounter groups, for staff, 228-232
Endicott, J., 233, 236, 264
Engelhardt, D. M., 160, 264
Engle, R. P., 118, 264
Erickson, G. D., 198, 265
Evaluation of treatment methods. See Research and evaluation

Fairweather, G. W., 46, 220, 265
Family involvement, 191-208
    and aftercare preparations, 204-208, 210-217
    and family-centered treatment, 200-201
    and goals of staff and family, 196
    and home visits by staff, 206-207, 215
    and information gathering, 193-197
    and medication of patient, 165-166
    and multiple family group therapy, 201-204
    and nuclear family therapy, 198-201
    and patient-centered treatment, 199
    and therapeutic program in hospital, 197-204
Ferster, C. B., 33, 100, 265
Fidler, G. S., 172, 265
Financial aspects of hospitalization, 9-10, 11, 18
Fischer, A., 153, 156, 265

Follow-up of patients from crisis intervention, 53-54
Forrest, F., 160, 161, 265
Forrest, I., 161, 265
Fox, J. V., 174, 265
Franks, C. M., 91, 265
Fromm-Reichmann, F., 16

Garber, B., 28, 140, 265
Gardner, J. M., 227, 265
Garlington, W. K., 80, 265
Gelfand, D. M., 106, 232, 265
Generalization process, in behavior modification, 89-91
Gericke, O. L., 80, 265
Glasser, N., 204, 269
Goffman, E., 3-4, 73, 265
Gonen, J. Y., 188, 265
Gorham, D. R., 154, 266
Gove, W. R., 212, 266
Gralnick, A., 28, 38, 140, 266
Grant, R. L., 71, 75, 124, 147, 232, 233, 235, 266
Greenblatt, M., 4, 118, 120, 266
Greenley, J. R., 29, 45, 71, 266
Grinspoon, L., 154, 266
Group design research, 238-239
Group pressure, in therapeutic community, 71-72
Group techniques
    in aftercare program, 221
    boundaries set in, 181
    educative model in, 180-181
    factors felt to be helpful in, 182-184
    "here and now" approach to, 185
    information sheet for, 257-259
    inpatients compared to outpatients in, 181, 183, 184
    multiple family group therapy, 201-204
    operational norms in, 181
    orientation sessions for, 181-182
    psychotherapy in, 179-186
    and qualities of hospital groups, 178-179
    reinforcers in, 184-185
    role-playing and psychodrama in, 188-190
    in staff sensitivity training, 228-232

in staffless groups, 186-187
in task groups, 187-188
in therapeutic commuunity, 62
Gruenberg, E. M., 31, 266
Guy, W., 233-236, 266

Haden, P., 162, 266
Hall, R. V., 95, 109, 242, 266
Hamilton, S. W., 6, 266
Handler, S. L., 194, 204, 267
Hansen, P. G., 186, 266
Hare, E. H., 159, 266
Harrow, M., 59, 178, 202, 204, 266, 267
Hartford Retreat, 8
Haun, P., 172, 174, 267
Havens, L. L., 154, 156, 157, 164, 267
Henderson, D., 15, 85, 267
Hersen, M., 30, 79, 83, 93, 94, 107, 267
Herz, M. I., 70, 75, 120, 267
Hes, J. P., 194, 201, 202, 203, 204, 267
Hilles, L., 123, 267
Historical aspects of hospital psychiatry, 5-20
and biological era, 13-15
and confinement, 5-7
and moral therapy, 7-10
and psychoanalysis, 15-16
and social psychiatry, 13, 17-20
and state hospital era, 10-13
History-taking
for activities therapy, 168-70
on admission, 124
family participation in, 193-197
Hogarty, G. E., 217, 267
Hollingshead, A. B., 18, 30, 118, 267
Home visits, by staff, 172, 206-207, 215
Hospital system, 126-138
and acting-up behavior, 131-135
disruptions of, 131-138
goals of, 127-129
limit setting in, 65, 132-134
and "special patient" syndrome, 135-137
specific treatment modalities in, 129-131
and violent behavior, 134-135
Houpt, J. L., 181, 221, 267

Housing programs, after discharge, 220-221

Imboden, J. B., 13, 267
Information gathering, See History-taking
Information sheet, for group therapy, 257-259
Institutionalization, historical aspects of, 5-7
Interaction-priming, 206-207
Intermediate-term hospital, 23
indications for, 122-123
organic therapy in, 30
and psychoanalysis, 28
and supportive psychotherapy, 27-28
and therapeutic community, 29
token economy in, 30
Irwin, D. S., 155, 159, 267

Jacobs, A., 110, 267
Jails, confinement in, 5
Johnson, C. A., 106, 267
Johnson, S. M., 93, 240, 267
Jones, M., 17, 25, 29, 43, 70, 71, 74, 228, 268
Jones, N., 36, 119, 268

Kadis, A. L., 186, 268
Kalogerakis, M. G., 134, 135, 268
Katz, R. C., 106, 107, 268
Kazdin, A. E., 80, 92, 95, 241, 268
Kernberg, O. F., 123, 268
Klein, D. F., 151, 268
Kole, C., 29, 268
Kramer, J. C., 162, 268
Krasner, L., 97, 262
Kraus, R., 167, 268
Kubie, L. S., 16, 268
Kupfer, D. J., 158, 233, 236, 268

Ladder system, in Tompkins-I, 60-61, 72
Laing, R. D., 4, 268
Lamb, H. R., 217, 268
Langsley, D. G., 120, 268
Laquer, H. P., 201, 203, 268
Lazare, A., 129, 268
LeBow, M. D., 37, 88, 91, 92, 95, 102, 104, 105, 109, 146, 195, 228, 243, 269

Lehmann, H. E., 157, 161, 165, 269
Leitenberg, H. W., 99, 269
Length of hospitalization, 23-24
  and crisis intervention, 51, 53
  and guidelines for admission,
    122-123
  in therapeutic community, 59, 70
  and token economy, 80, 81, 83
Levin, E. C., 201, 204, 269
Lewis, F. A., 4, 269
Lewis, J. C., 202, 204, 269
Liberman, R., 205, 269
Lichtenberg, J. B., 118, 269
Lidz, T., 17, 192, 269
Lieb, J., 27, 50, 269
Limit setting, 65, 127, 132-134
Lindemann, E., 24, 269
Lindsley, O. R., 79, 269
Linn, E. L., 119, 269
Linn, L., 27, 269
Linn, L. S., 28, 119, 120, 269
Lion, J. R., 134, 135, 269
Lipsius, L. H., 235, 269
Lloyd, K. E., 30, 81, 269
Long-term hospitals, 24
  custodial care in, 30-31
  indications for, 123
  and psychoanalysis, 28-29
  therapeutic community in, 29
  token economy in, 29-30
Lorr, M., 236-269
Lucero, R. J., 110, 269
Ludwig, A. M., 45, 73, 147, 270

MacDonald, J. M., 132, 135, 270
MacLean Hospital, 12
Main, T. F., 25, 44, 135, 228, 270
Malamud, W., 7, 12, 270
Maletzky, B. M., 232, 266
Mann, H., 9
Marohn, R. C., 133, 270
Martin, P. L., 85, 95, 272
Maxmen, J. S., 22, 31, 45, 53, 59,
  118, 124, 183, 270
May, P. R. A., 154, 239, 270
Medications, 26, 30, 151-166
  and collaboration of patient,
    156-159
  and drug schedule charts, 159
  guidelines for use of, 153-155

historical aspects of, 14
in intermediate-term hospital, 30
resistance to, 159-166
side effects check list, 158
side effects of, 158, 162
staff attitudes toward, 155-156
staff familiarity with, 152-153
and symptom chart use, 157-158
Mendel, W. M., 4, 118, 119, 270
Menninger, K., 16
Menninger, W., 16, 28, 270
Menninger Clinic, 16
Mental health centers, development
  of, 18-19
Mental illness, theories of, 6, 7, 12,
  13-14, 38-39
Michael, J., 101, 262
Milieu therapy. See Therapeutic
  community
Miller, E. J., 126, 270
Minuchin, S., 196, 270
Miron, N. B., 110, 270
Mitchell, S. W., 12, 270
Moos, R. H., 41, 270
Moral therapy, historical aspects of,
  7-10
Moreno, J. L., 178, 188, 270
Morris, N., 106, 271
Mosey, A. C., 169, 270
Muller, D. J., 173, 271
Muller, J. J., 36, 271
Multiple family group therapy,
  201-204
Myers, A., 12
Myers, K., 29, 271

Neve, H. K., 159, 271
Norton, N. M., 201, 271

O'Brien, F., 206, 211, 271
Operants, in token economy, 88-89
Organic disorders, and mental
  illness, 13-15
Organic therapies. See Electrocon-
  vulsive therapy; Medications
Outpatient care,
  historical aspects of, 13
  reference to, 217-219
Overall, J. E., 236, 271

Panyon, M., 106, 107, 271
Pao, P. -N., 118, 271
Pasamanick, B., 120, 271
Pasternak, S. A., 134, 269
Patients
    authority relationships with staff,
        74-77
    bond with staff culture, in thera-
        peutic communuity, 73-74
    as collaborators in drug treat-
        ment, 156-159
    meetings with staff, in thera-
        peutic community, 60-65, 75
    as rehabilitative agents, 45-46,
        58, 69-72, 73
    resistance to medication, 159-166
    in staffless groups, 186-187
    therapeutic responsibilities in
        group therapy, 180-181
    token economy affecting, 80
Patterson, G. R., 205, 228, 271
Paul, G. L., 80, 95, 271
Pavlov, I. P., 88
Pennsylvania Hospital, 7
Peterson, D. P., 162, 271
Phipps Clinic, 13
Pierce, W. D., 231, 271
Pinsker, H., 57, 58, 271
Polak, P., 27, 271
Polansky, N. A., 190, 271
Poor houses, confinement in, 6
Poser, E. G., 228, 271
Pratt, J. H., 177, 271
Premack, D., 92, 272
Problem-oriented record, 233-236
Psychiatric Status Schedule, 53
Psychodrama, 188-190
Psychotherapy, 24-25, 139-144
    group, 179-186
    historical aspects of, 15-16
    individual psychotherapy,
        140-144
    in intermediate-term hospitals,
        29
    in long-term hospitals, 28-29
    supportive, 24-25, 27

Querido, A., 4, 272
Rapport, S., 119, 270
Raskin, D. E., 29, 70, 272
Ratic of staff to patients, 27

Reactive environment, 33-46
    and adjustment in community, 41
    admission process in, 117-125
    and aftercare preparations, 43,
        209-222
    and evaluation of behavioral
        functioning, 42
    and hospital system, 126-138
    patient's role in, 45-46, 58, 69-72,
        73
    and sources of change, 43-46
    staff role in, 43-45
    therapeutic settings in, 41
Record keeping, 232-237
    goal-oriented record, 235-236
    problem-oriented record, 233-236
    standardized inter-connected
        systems in, 236-237
Redlich, F. C., 18, 229, 272
Re-entry group, 221
Referral of patients to outside
    therapists, 217-219
Rehabilitation, 38
    patients as agents for, 45-46, 58,
        69-72, 73
Reinforcers for behavior modifica-
    tion, 103-105, 147
    family involvement in, 196-197
    in group psychotherapy, 184-185
    for patients in token economy,
        87-88, 92, 97-98, 100-101, 103
    for staff in token economy,
        105-108
    in therapeutic community, 72
    See also Behavior Modification
        procedure
Relatives. See Family involvement
Research and evaluation, 237-243
    group design, 238-239
    multiple baseline design, 242-243
    reversal design, 240-242
    single-subject design, 239-240
Resistance of patients to medica-
    tion, 159-166
Reynolds, G. S., 88, 272
Responsibility, sharing of, in thera-
    peutic community, 72
Restraints, use of, 7-8
Rice, A. K., 231, 272
Rinsley, D. B., 28, 140, 272
Rogoff, M. -L., 275

Role-playing techniques, 188-190
and training of staff, 227
Rosenberg, S. D., 31, 272
Rosenzweig, N., 27, 272
Rothaus, P., 186, 272
Rothman, D. J., 5, 6, 272
Rubenstein, R., 16, 38, 272
Rural areas, facilities in, 52-53
Rush, B., 7

Sadoff, R. L., 219, 272
Sager, C. J., 45, 57, 198, 229, 272
Sanders, D. H., 220, 272
Sarwer-Foner, G. J., 155, 272
Schaefer, H. H., 78, 85, 95, 147, 272
Schein, E. H., 180, 272
Schulberg, H., 49, 272
Schwartz, M. S., 17, 43, 228, 273
Scoles, P. E., 85, 267
Sensitivity training for staff,
228-232
Shanfield, S., 239, 273
Sherman, J. A., 241, 273
Short-term hospitals, 23
and crisis intervention, 27, 49-55
indications for, 122
and patients as rehabilitative
agents, 45
and supportive psychotherapy,
27-28
Side effects check list, 158
Skinner, B. F., 85, 87, 96, 110, 273
Slavson, S. R., 178, 180, 273
Smith, C. G., 120, 273
Smith, R. C., 100, 144, 147, 273
Social psychiatry, historical aspects
of, 13, 17-20
Social reinforcers,
in therapeutic community, 71-72
in token economy, 98-99
Solomon, L. N., 178, 273
Solow, C., 52, 273
Spadoni, A. J., 74, 273
"Special patient" syndrome, 135-137
Spitzer, R. L., 53, 233, 236, 273
Staff
attitudes toward medications,
155-156
authority relationships with
patients, 74-77
bond with patient culture, 73-74

in crisis intervention, 51, 54
effective utilization of, 43-45
familiarity with medications,
152-153
home visits by, 172, 206-207, 215
knowledge of patient's behavior
pattern, 42
meetings with patients, 62-65, 76
ratio to patients, 26, 53, 60
reinforcers for, in token economy,
105-108
sensitivity training for, 228-232
in therapeutic community, 68-70,
72-75
in token economy, 78, 93, 105-108
training of, 226-232
Staffless groups, 186-187
Stancer, H. C., 118, 273
Stanton, A. H., 17, 43, 44, 73, 228,
232, 273
State hospitals, historical background of, 10-13
Sullivan, H. S., 16, 17, 273
Supportive psychotherapy, 24-25, 27
Sutherland, J. D., 180, 185, 273
Symptom chart, use of, 157-158
Szasz, T. S., 4, 273

Task groups, 187-188
Therapeutic community, 25, 57-77
advisory board in, 60-62, 69, 74
authority relationships in, 74-77
basic principles of, 69-72
and bond between staff and patient cultures, 73-74
characteristics of patients in,
59-60
confidentiality in, 71, 73
emergency sessions in, 65
expectations in, 71
group pressure in, 72
group sessions in, 62
historical aspects of, 8-9- 17
in intermediate-term hospitals,
29
ladder system in, 60-62, 72
in long-term hospitals, 29
patient-staff meetings in, 62-65,
75
and patients as change agents,
45, 58, 69-72, 73

rewards and punishments in, 72
shared responsibility in, 72
staff role in, 66-69
treatment program in, 60-63
typical schedule in, 67
value system in, 73-74
Thomas, C. S., 50, 273
Thomson, L., 99, 269
Time-sampling, in token economy, 95-96
Token economy, 18, 25-26, 78-113
  behavioristic foundations of, 108-113
  contingencies in, 97
  and control of behavior, 111- 112
  and defining of behavior, 86, 109
  deprivation in, 110-111
  and describing patients, 108-109
  direction of change in, 86-87
  effects on patients, 80
  evaluative data in, 94
  examples of, 81-85
  follow-up data in, 94-95
  immediate reinforcement in, 97-98
  in intermediate-term hospital, 30
  in long-term hospital, 29-30
  measurable products in, 109-110
  operants in, 88-89
  and patients as rehabilitative agents, 45, 144-145
  and post-hospital functioning, 80, 94-95, 107
  recording of behavior in, 91-96
  reinforcing staff performance in, 105-108
  social reinforcers in, 98-99
  staff responsibilities in, 78, 93
  target behavior in, 83, 86, 92
  techniques used in, 100-105
  terms and meanings in, 85-91
  time-sampling in, 95-96
  tokens in, 96-100
  See also Behavior modification procedures
Tompkins-I, 58-76, 186, 239, 245-256
Training of staff, 226-232
  sensitivity sessions for, 228-232
Treatment modalities, 24-26
  activities therapy, 167-176
  and admission procedures, 117-125
  behavior modification in, 36-40, 144-149
  crisis intervention in, 49-55
  evaluation of, 237-243
  family involvement in, 191-208
  group techniques in, 177-190
  and hospital system, 129-131
  medications in, 151-166
  multiple techniques in, 40
  and planning for aftercare, 209-222
  psychotherapy in, 139-144
  tailoring of, 40-43
  in therapeutic community, 57-77
  and token economy, 79-113
Tucker, G. J., 36, 39, 40, 45, 70, 201, 203, 273
Types of hospital units, 18, 21-31

Uhlenhuth, E. H., 155, 273
Underwood, W. J., 229, 274
Upper, D., 102, 274

Vaillant, G. E., 122, 274
Violent behavior, control of, 127, 134-135

Wachspress, M., 172, 274
Wanklin, J. M., 118, 274
Ward Atmosphere Scale, 231
Weed, L. L., 233, 235, 274
Weintraub, W., 119, 131, 274
Weisman, G., 27, 50, 51, 52, 274
Whitaker, C. A., 229, 274
Whitely, J. S., 29, 274
Wilmer, H. A., 17, 58, 274
Winer, B. J., 239, 274
Wolf, A., 186, 274
Wolpe, J., 144, 274
Wood, E. C., 118, 274
Worcester State Hospital, 8, 9
Work houses, confinement in, 6
Wynne, L. C., 192, 274

Yale Psychiatric Institute, 16
Yalom, I. D., 178, 183, 185, 274

Zeitlyn, B. B., 58, 274